HOD
LIB   P9-DZA-121

A HANDBOOK OF BIOETHICS TERMS

HODGES UNIVERSITY
LIBRARY - NAPLES

A HANDBOOK OF BIOETHICS TERMS

James B. Tubbs Jr.

Georgetown University Press ∽ Washington, D.C.

Georgetown University Press, Washington, D.C.
www.press.georgetown.edu
© 2009 by Georgetown University Press. All rights reserved. No part of
this book may be reproduced or utilized in any form or by any means,
electronic or mechanical, including photocopying and recording, or by
any information storage and retrieval system, without permission in
writing from the publisher.

Library of Congress Cataloging-in-Publication Data

Tubbs, James B.
   A handbook of bioethics terms / James B. Tubbs Jr.
      p. ; cm.
   Includes bibliographical references and index.
   ISBN 978-1-58901-259-2 (pbk. : alk. paper)
   1. Medical ethics—Handbooks, manuals, etc. 2. Bioethics—Handbooks,
manuals, etc. 3. Medical ethics—Dictionaries. 4. Bioethics—Dictionaries.
I. Title.
   [DNLM: 1. Bioethics—Dictionary—English. W 13 T884h 2008]
   R725.5.T83 2008
   174.2—dc22

                                                      2008033987

  ∞ This book is printed on acid-free paper meeting the requirements of
the American National Standard for Permanence in Paper for Printed
Library Materials.

15 14 13 12 11 10 09   9 8 7 6 5 4 3 2
First printing

Printed in the United States of America

Contents

Preface

For many centuries physicians have reflected upon the moral virtues and obligations of their profession, and philosophers and theologians have analyzed, debated, and opined about particular moral dilemmas and choices in health care such as abortion, mutilation of the body for therapeutic purposes, and acceptance or rejection of life-prolonging treatment. Thus, it might be fair to say that the modern discipline of reflection upon ethical aspects of biomedicine began as a subset or focused application of those disciplines. Yet the contemporary discipline of bioethics began to emerge in the 1960s as a broader, more interdisciplinary phenomenon, built upon dialogue not simply among physicians, theologians, and philosophers but including other health professionals, natural scientists, social scientists, legal scholars, and policymakers.

The term "bioethics" was first used in the early 1970s by biologists who were concerned about ethical implications of genetic and ecological interventions, but it was soon applied to all aspects of "biomedical ethics," including health care delivery, research, and public policy. From its modern beginnings, then, the discipline of bioethics has been focused on knowledge and ethical reflection from multiple disciplinary vantage points, recognizing the value of ethical wisdom from varied perspectives as well as the commonality of many issues and dilemmas we face. In his introduction to the revised edition of the *Encyclopedia of Bioethics* (New York: MacMillan, 1995), editor in chief Warren T. Reich defines bioethics as "the systematic study of the moral dimensions— including moral vision, decisions, conduct, and policies—of the life sciences and health care, employing a variety of ethical methodologies in an interdisciplinary setting."

Of course, this multidisciplinary focus can also present significant challenges for the education and preparation of any single individual aspiring to be a "bioethicist." In an article titled "Bioethics as a Discipline" in the very first issue of the *Hastings Center Studies* (1973), Daniel Callahan suggested a formidable ideal list of necessary ingredients in the training of a bioethicist:

> . . . sociological understanding of the medical and biological communities; psychological understanding of the kinds of needs felt by researchers and clinicians, patients and physicians, and the varieties of pressures to which they are subject; historical understanding of the sources of the regnant value theories and common practices; requisite scientific training; awareness of and facility with the usual methods of ethical analysis as understood in the philosophical and theological communities—and no less a full awareness of the limitations of those methods when applied to actual cases; and, finally, personal exposure to the kinds of ethical problems which arise in medicine and biology. (*Hastings Center Studies* 1, no. 1 [1973]: 73.)

Callahan himself recognized that this constituted an "impossible list of demands" for any individual. At the same time, however, it is clear that the perspectives and knowledge bases he lists are certainly necessary aspects of the kind of analysis and reflection that must be undertaken within the discipline. Put in other words, the work of the discipline of bioethics is impossible without input from the knowledge and wisdom of many other disciplines. Bioethics is, then, inherently a function of disciplines in dialogue.

Effective dialogue, however, requires not only intentionality and receptivity but also the fundamental tools of communication, including commonly understood language, vocabulary, figures of speech, and so on. And one of the realities of interdisciplinary, interprofessional dialogue is that, even within a common language system, most individual disciplines, guilds, or professions have developed their own unique vocabularies or have attached new definitions to commonly used terms. Thus, one possible barrier to fully effective interdisciplinary communication of the sort necessary in bioethics is the wide array of terminologies (or alternate definitions) not shared among all participants. The primary purpose of this little handbook, then, is to assuage in some small way the "vocabulary gap" encountered by so many students of bioethics.

One inspiration for this project was theologian Van A. Harvey's *A Handbook of Theological Terms*, first published in 1964. Harvey's aim was to help make theological discourse more accessible to interested laypersons by providing them with an understanding of some of the traditional and technical vocabulary of theology, especially systematic and philosophical theology. Yet Harvey was attempting to make the discourse of only one discipline more accessible in this way; the problem I am trying to address is the multiplicity of vocabularies faced not only by those outside the disciplines involved in bioethical reflection but also by those in each of the dialoguing disciplines who are not familiar with the vocabularies of others.

My approach here grows out of experiences of frustration— my own and my students'—in navigating technical jargon at many levels. As a college student I majored in biology but was also very interested in the humanities. I was not entirely convinced that I was living between the very different "two

cultures" (of the sciences and the humanities) described by
C. P. Snow, but I was very much aware of the different
vocabularies with which I had to communicate. During and
after college I held several patient-contact positions in health
care institutions and was challenged to master yet another
vocabulary to function well in that context. Then, in a
graduate program in ethics in a department of religious studies, I was faced with yet other vocabularies as necessary tools
of comprehension and discourse. Now I teach courses in
health care ethics for students from many different academic
programs and disciplines, and I am very much aware of the
struggles many of them face in dealing with the discipline-
specific jargon in some of the articles they read (or even in
what they hear from me). In addition, my service on various
hospital ethics committees constantly reminds me how much
I do not yet know about the vocabularies of clinical medicine, nursing, and research.

This handbook, then, is intended primarily as a help for
those facing unfamiliar terminology in their exploration of
bioethics literature or in their participation in bioethics discourse—students in health care ethics courses, for example,
or members of institutional ethics committees. It is intended
to be relatively brief and handy, not exhaustive; it is not a
dictionary or an encyclopedia. It is simply a glossary-style
handbook of terms, expressions, and titles that may be
encountered in the literature of bioethics. Some entries are
very brief while others provide more interpretive background
or context for the entry term. Some entries—a minority—
also include references to other published works that provide
broader explication and analysis of that particular entry term.
Each entry term is printed in bold type; within the text of
each entry, bold type may be used to designate a term for
which a separate entry occurs elsewhere in the handbook. In
an attempt to use gender-neutral language, he/she, his/her,

and all variants of these terms have been used in alternating entries, except where gender-specific terms are appropriate.

Of course, any project of this sort is also a glaring advertisement of the author's own subjectivity and experiential limitations in selecting terms for inclusion (or exclusion). I must confess that I continue to second-guess my own selections nearly every day! And I am certain that many readers will be disappointed that I have not provided a description or explanation for some term about which they are curious. Yet, my hope is that the commentary provided in this handbook will be useful enough, and to enough people, to justify its creation.

Acknowledgments

This book grew out of a conversation I had several years ago with Richard Brown, director of Georgetown University Press. I had long recognized a need among my health care ethics students for some kind of resource for understanding the terminologies of clinical medicine and of theology and philosophy. But the form this project has taken was Richard's original idea—and I thank him for that, not only because the handbook that has resulted may be useful to others but also because the process of researching and writing it has been a most enjoyable exercise in self-education. Richard has also been a constant source of encouragement, good humor, and good advice. Others, too, have offered useful suggestions, criticisms, and assistance. A semester research leave from the University of Detroit Mercy allowed me to get this project well under way. My colleague David Nantais read the first draft of the manuscript and offered valuable suggestions for additions and revisions. Two anonymous reviewers for Georgetown University Press also provided very helpful critiques and suggestions, some general and some very specific, and I have been able to incorporate most of their suggestions into the handbook's final form. To all these contributors I am most grateful. Their inputs have made this book a better and more useful work. Any significant omissions or mistakes that remain are, however, my own.

Bioethics Terms

❧ **A** ❧

Abortifacient: A chemical or other substance that induces abortion.

Abortion: In traditional clinical terminology, expulsion from the uterus of an embryo or fetus before it is viable (i.e., developmentally capable of independent existence). While *spontaneous* abortion (also known as "miscarriage") is a common occurrence, the term "abortion" is most often used to refer to *induced* abortion—that is, abortion brought on intentionally via medical or surgical means (in contemporary usage it can refer to the removal of the fetus from the uterus after the point of probable viability as well). The practice of induced abortion is believed to predate recorded history, and some of the earliest medically related historical documents (e.g., Chinese, Egyptian, Greek, and Roman) refer to the practice. Debates about the morality of abortion also have an ancient pedigree and through the centuries have focused on such concerns as maternal well-being, openness to or control of fertility, beliefs about the actualized or potential personhood of the fetus, societal circumstances, and so on. In the United States, legal regulation (and then prohibition) of abortion practices began to be exercised by the states in the early nineteenth century, and by the 1880s most abortion procedures had been legally proscribed throughout the country. In 1973, however, the U.S. Supreme Court issued its **Roe v. Wade** decision, affirming women's reproductive liberty-based right to choose abortion in the first or second trimester of pregnancy; the state's interest in protecting maternal health, which would allow for regulation of how and where abortions are performed during the second trimester; and the state's interest in protecting the potentiality of human life, which would allow for legal proscription of abortion in the third trimester unless the pregnancy threatens the mother's life or health. Abortion procedures currently practiced in the United States vary according to the stage of pregnancy. In the first trimester, abortion may be induced by surgical or medical means. Suction aspiration (also called "suction curettage" or "vacuum aspiration"), the most widely used abortion method, involves suction removal of uterine contents through a flexible tube introduced via the cervix; it is usually performed between six and thirteen weeks of gestation (counting from the woman's last menstrual period). Medical abortion, usually performed up until weeks seven to nine, involves use of drugs such as methotrexate or **mifepristone** (previously referred to as **RU-486**) to cause fetal death, combined with a contraction-inducing drug such as misoprostol. In the second trimester, dilation and curettage (D&C) and dilation and evacuation (D&E) involve dilation of the cervix followed by removal of fetus and placenta via surgical instruments or vacuum suction, or both. In another, now-rare form of second- and third-trimester abortion known as induction abortion, strong salt or other chemical solutions are introduced into the uterus, causing fetal death, after which uterine contractions are chemically induced. In recent years much public controversy has arisen about another form of late (after twenty-one weeks' gestation) abortion called dilation and extraction (D&X or Intact D&X), also referred to as partial-birth abortion. This procedure involves cervical dilation followed by partial delivery of the intact fetus feet first; then a sharp instrument is inserted into the back of the fetus's head and the brain is suctioned before delivery is completed. One other rarely employed abortion procedure is the hysterotomy abortion, in which the fetus is removed by making an incision in the pregnant woman's abdomen and into the uterus; this is essentially an early Caesarian section delivery, albeit not resulting in live birth. (See also **therapeutic abortion**)

Acquired immune deficiency syndrome (AIDS):   A syndrome in which the body's immune system fails, leading to serious opportunistic infections. (See **human immunodeficiency virus**)

Active euthanasia: Sometimes referred to as "mercy killing." Active euthanasia involves the use of drugs or other lethal means to cause the peaceful death of the individual being euthanized. (See **euthanasia**)

Act-utilitarianism: A form of moral reasoning in which judgment about the "right" thing to do is based upon a calculus of overall predicted good and bad consequences for each possible course of action in that particular situation. (See **utilitarianism**)

Adult stem cells: See **stem cells**

Advance directive [for health care]:   A declaration, usually written, in which an individual describes the forms of medical treatment he wishes to receive, or designates another individual to make those treatment decisions on his behalf, should the directive's author lose decision-making capacity at some future date. In the United States, two major types of advance directive have gained widespread usage and legal recognition: the living will and the durable power of attorney for health care. A living will allows its author to define the types of medical treatment that he would choose to receive, as well as those that would be unwanted (and under what conditions), in the event the author becomes unable to choose or communicate those treatment choices in the future. In other words, the living will is a form of prospective consent to, or rejection of, specified forms of treatment—quite often life-extending treatments. Conversely, a durable power of attorney for health care allows an author to designate a particular person or persons to act as his health care proxy for treatment choices, in the event that the author becomes incapable of forming or expressing those choices in the future. In other words, a durable power of attorney represents the author's prospective consent to those forms of treatment chosen on his behalf by the designated proxy or advocate.

AI (also AID and AIH):   See **artificial insemination**

AIDS: See **acquired immune deficiency syndrome; human immunodeficiency virus**

Allele: One of a number of possible **DNA (deoxyribonucleic acid)** segments occupying a particular location on a **chromosome,** usually comprising a **gene.** For example, if hair color is determined by a particular DNA sequence (or gene) at a particular location on a particular chromosome, then the gene coding for brown hair and the gene coding for blonde hair are alleles of one another. Humans are **diploid** organisms whose **somatic cells** contain two full sets of chromosomes (one set from each parent); thus, each somatic cell has two alleles for each chromosome location (one on each paired chromosome). If both alleles at a given location are the same for each of the chromosomes in the pair, then the individual is said to be **homozygous** for that particular gene at that location. If the two alleles differ, then the individual is **heterozygous** for that gene.

Allocation: Distribution in the form of apportionment or allotment among persons or groups. At the broad social/political/economic level, macroallocation decisions apportion or allocate resources (usually funding) for particular kinds of goods or services and determine the methods of their distribution. For instance, federal funding for Medicare, the Veteran's Administration (VA) hospital system, or the National Parks Service requires macroallocation decisions. Microallocation decisions apportion or allot among persons particular resources that are scarce (either naturally or because of previous macroallocation decisions). Distribution of scarce cadaver organs for transplant among the many potential recipients is an example of microallocation. The term **"rationing"** is sometimes employed as a synonym for microallocation, although some commentators also use that term to refer to certain macroallocation decisions as well.

Allograft (homograft):   Tissue or organ taken from a donor organism and transplanted into a recipient organism of the same species but of different genetic makeup, thus requiring suppression of the recipient's immune system to prevent rejection of the graft. (See **transplantation, organ and tissue**)

Allopathic medicine: Term sometimes used to refer to conventional, traditional, or prevailing medical practice (in contrast to homeopathic or osteopathic medicine). The term was introduced in the mid-nineteenth century by C. F. S. Hahnemann, the founder of homeopathy, to distinguish that practice from the "usual" practice of medicine at that time, which he termed "allopathy."

Amniocentesis: A technique for **prenatal diagnosis** performed by inserting a hollow needle through the pregnant woman's abdomen into the uterus and withdrawing a sample of fluid from the amniotic sac surrounding the fetus. The sample fluid, which also contains loosed fetal cells, can be tested to diagnose many fetal characteristics and conditions, such as gender, fetal lung development, chromosomal abnormalities (e.g., **Down syndrome**), inherited metabolic disorders (e.g., **Tay-Sachs disease** or **Lesch-Nyhan syndrome**), neural tube defects (e.g., **spina bifida, anencephaly**), and suspected problems such as infection or maternal–fetal Rh incompatibility. Amniocentesis is the most widely used method of prenatal diagnosis.

Anemia: A condition (with many causes) in which the body's blood contains fewer than normal red blood cells or the red blood cells contain insufficient oxygen-carrying hemoglobin molecules.

Anencephaly: A condition caused by failure of the forward end of the neural tube to fully close, so that the infant is born without a forebrain (or cerebral hemispheres) and with remaining brain tissue often not covered by skull or skin. (See **neural tube defect**)

Aneuploidy: The condition of having more or less than the normal **diploid** number of chromosomes in the cell nucleus (in humans, twenty-three pairs of autosomal chromosomes and two sex chromosomes—also called euploidy). Aneuploidy is the most frequently observed form of cytogenetic abnormality. In monosomy, one of a pair of chromosomes is missing. So, for example, "monosomy 12" would mean that only one chromosome 12 is present in the nucleus of each cell, or, as in Turner's syndrome, only one sex chromosome is present. In trisomy, three chromosomes of a particular type are present, as in Down syndrome (Trisomy 21), Edward's syndrome (Trisomy 18), Patau's syndrome (Trisomy 13), Klinefelter's syndrome (XXY), or XYY syndrome. In tetraploidy, four chromosomes of a particular type would be present. (Trisomies and tetraploidies would both be polyploid conditions.) Chromosomal aneuploidies may lead to prenatal or early infant mortality or may cause birth defects, infertility, mental retardation, or other genetic syndromes. A majority of prenatal diagnostic procedures are chosen and performed to detect chromosomal aneuploidies.

Animation: Literally, the process of taking on life, or becoming alive. In the history of Western philosophy and theology (especially since Aristotle), however, the term "animation" (together with the roughly synonymous terms "hominization" and "ensoulment") has often been used to refer to the process within human embryology in which the product of conception takes on a rational soul and thus becomes a fully human being. Aristotle believed that the human embryo/fetus takes on human form—that is, becomes "animated" or "ensouled"—at forty days after conception (for the male) or eighty to ninety days after conception (for the female). This view, later reflected in the works of Christian theologians Augustine and Aquinas and apparently dominant in medieval Roman Catholic theology, has been termed delayed animation or mediate animation. In contrast, immediate animation/hominization refers to the belief that the human soul is present from the moment of conception. Theories of delayed animation/hominization have been expressed in the history of Islamic theology as well as Christian theology; however, more recent (late nineteenth and twentieth century) official teachings within both theological traditions have tended to reject the notion of delayed animation.

Antibodies: Proteins produced by the immune system that attach to and cause the neutralization of **antigens** that invade the body.

Antigen (or immunogen):   A foreign molecule (pollen, for example) or a protein molecule on the surface of an infectious agent (bacteria or virus) that provokes a response from the body's immune system. The presence of antigens elicits the production of protein **antibodies** that specifically attach to and deactivate or destroy the invasive antigens.

Apgar score: A test designed to measure and report aspects of a newborn infant's physical condition and vital functions. Developed by anesthesiologist Virginia Apgar in 1952, the test represents an assessment of five physiological factors represented by the acronym APGAR: activity (muscle tone); pulse (heart rate); grimace (responsiveness or "reflex irritability"); appearance (skin coloration); and respiration (breathing rate). Each of these five factors is scored on a scale of 0 to 2; thus a combined or total Apgar score ranges between 0 (immediate resuscitation needed) and 10 (the best possible condition). The five factors are usually scored at one minute after birth and then again at five minutes after birth. In cases of infant distress and low Apgar scores, the test may be repeated at 10, 15, or 20 minutes after birth. The Apgar score was not designed to predict a baby's long-term outcome, health, behavior, or intellectual status; however, low scores measured at repeated intervals have been shown to be predictive of high rates of neonatal morbidity (illness) and mortality (death).

Applied ethics: A term referring to the application of ethical theory, ethical reasoning, or ethical perspective to particular areas of human life and activity—for example, business ethics, legal ethics, health care ethics, or pastoral ethics—or to particular problems, such as the moral issue of abortion or of warfare. The term "practical ethics" is often used as a synonym for applied ethics. (See **ethics**)

Aretaic ethics (or aretology):   See **virtue ethics**

ART: See **assisted reproductive technology**

Artificial insemination (AI):   A procedure in which a man's sperm is introduced into a woman's vagina, uterus, or fallopian tubes by artificial means (rather than by sexual intercourse) to facilitate fertilization and pregnancy. In AIH (artificial insemination by husband), the woman's partner's sperm is used, whereas sperm from a donor is used in AID (artificial insemination by donor). Types of AI also differ with regard to the location of insemination in the female reproductive tract: intrauterine (in the uterus); intracervical (in the cervical canal); intrafollicular (in the ovarian follicle); and intratubal (in the fallopian tubes).

Artificial womb/placenta: See **ectogenesis**

Assisted reproductive technology (ART):   All treatments or procedures involving the handling or manipulation of both ova (eggs) and sperm for the purpose of helping a woman to become pregnant. (This definition, as employed by the U.S. Centers for Disease Control, would not include treatments or procedures in which only sperm are handled, as in artificial insemination, or procedures in which a woman's production of ova is stimulated but without the intention of ova retrieval.) ART usually involves surgical removal of ova from a woman's ovaries, combining them with sperm in the laboratory, and then returning them to the woman's body (or another woman's body). Six main types of ART are employed in the United States. The most common, **in vitro fertilization (IVF),** involves combining surgically retrieved ova with donated sperm in a laboratory dish, after which the fertilized embryo is transferred to the woman's uterus through the cervix. In intracytoplasmic sperm injection (ICSI), a single sperm cell is injected into a retrieved ovum, after which it is placed in the woman's uterus or fallopian tube. This is often a successful form of treatment in cases where infertility has been due to the man's impaired sperm. **Gamete intrafallopian transfer (GIFT)** involves mixing ova and sperm together in a laboratory dish, then injecting the mixture via a laparoscope into the woman's fallopian tubes where fertilization takes place. Zygote intrafallopian transfer (ZIFT) is like GIFT, but fertilization is allowed to happen in the laboratory dish, after which the resulting zygotes (pre-embryos) are transferred to the fallopian tubes (through which they will travel to the uterus for implantation). Yet another form of ART involves using ova retrieved from a female donor, which are then mixed with the recipient woman's partner's sperm, after which the resultant embryos are implanted into the recipient's uterus. Finally, **surrogate gestation** is a procedure in which a female "surrogate" carries to term an embryo placed into her uterus following from the fertilization of ova from the "adoptive" woman (or a donor) by sperm from the "adoptive" woman's partner (or a donor). In this arrangement, the "surrogate" agrees to give the baby to the "adoptive" parent(s) at birth.

Assisted suicide: See **suicide**

Autograft: A transplant of tissue from one part of a person's body into another part of her body. (See **transplantation, organ and tissue**)

Autoimmune disease: A disease or disorder in which the body's own cells are mistakenly identified as foreign material by the body and therefore attacked by the body's immune defense system, causing cellular and tissue damage or death.

Examples include multiple sclerosis, type 1 diabetes mellitus, rheumatoid arthritis, Crohn's disease, and systemic lupus erythematosus.

Autonomy: Literally, "self-law" or "self-rule" (from the Greek *autos*, or "self," and *nomos*, "rule" or "law"). The term has been applied historically both to the self-government of political communities and to the **self-determination** of individuals. Moral autonomy refers to an individual's free recognition and acceptance of those moral norms or action guides that will govern her attitudes and behaviors (as opposed to **heteronomy,** or moral governance according to norms established and imposed by authorities outside the self). Immanuel Kant famously identified autonomous moral agents as self-legislating, that is, as freely acting according to the categorical imperative (always following those maxims one would will to be universal moral laws). Heteronomous agents, on the other hand, act according to principles of action derived not from the categorical imperative but from other considerations (e.g., goals or consequences of actions) and sources (e.g., passion, desire, the will and command of others). (See Immanuel Kant, *Groundwork of the Metaphysic of Morals,* trans. H. J. Paton [New York: Harper and Row, 1964],) In the ethics of health care, respect for individual autonomy is generally understood to mean respect for various forms of self-determination and individual control over one's own body. Thus it presupposes that the individual whose autonomy is to be respected has the capacity to form and express choices on her own behalf. It also presupposes the possibility of, and requires respect for, her liberty, that is, freedom of thought, self-directed action, and self-regarding choice, including the freedom to give or withhold consent to medical treatment or research participation for oneself. Respect for autonomy is also viewed as the ground or basis for several other patient-regarding norms as well, including respect for privacy (of information, personal space, decisions, and personal property) and maintenance of confidentiality (of patient-related information). Furthermore, because any true exercise of autonomy via voluntary, informed consent would require prior disclosure and comprehension of accurate and complete information, respect for autonomy may also be seen as a foundation for the norm of truthfulness in the disclosure of patient-centered information. (See, for example, Beauchamp and Childress, *Principles of Biomedical Ethics,* 6th ed. [New York: Oxford University Press, 2009], especially chapters 4 and 8.)

Autosomal disorder: A genetic disease or disorder whose causative gene is located on an autosome—a non–sex-selecting chromosome. Thus, autosomal disorders may be inherited by children of either sex. In an autosomal dominant disorder (e.g., Huntington's disease), the disorder or disease is manifest (expressed) in the offspring when the causative gene is inherited from either parent. In an autosomal recessive disorder (e.g., **sickle cell disease**), the causative gene must be inherited from both parents for the disease or disorder to be manifest in the offspring. Any offspring inheriting the causative gene from only one parent would be a "carrier" for that autosomal disorder.

B

"Baby Doe" regulations: Popular name applied to a series of federal regulations addressing the medical treatment of handicapped infants. The rules were in part a reaction to the 1982 Indiana case of "Baby Doe," an infant with tracheo-esophogeal fistula who was allowed to die without corrective surgery because he also had Down syndrome. In response, the Reagan administration issued guidelines for all hospitals receiving federal funding, reminding them that the Rehabilitation Act of 1973 would require maximal life-prolonging treatment of all infants, regardless of handicap, unless the treatment itself was medically contraindicated. These guidelines also established what became known as "Baby Doe Hotlines," publicized telephone numbers by which hospital employees could notify federal regulators of suspected violations of the published treatment guidelines. While several parts of these first regulations were overturned by federal courts, the U.S. Congress soon passed the similarly aimed "Child Abuse Prevention and Treatment Act of 1984." This law specifies that all infants should be provided "appropriate nutrition, hydration and medication" and that life-prolonging treatment may be withheld only if the infant is "chronically and irreversibly comatose," if provision of the treatment would be ineffective in correcting the infant's life-threatening conditions or otherwise "futile" in terms of the infant's survival, or if provision of the treatment would be "virtually futile" and "inhumane" under the infant's particular circumstances. (See, e.g., L. M. Kopelman, "Are the 21-Year-Old

Baby Doe Rules Misunderstood or Mistaken?" *Pediatrics* 115 [2005]: 797–802.)

Baby M case: 1988 New Jersey Supreme Court case (*In re Baby M,* 537 A.2D. 1227 [N.J. 1988]) concerning the legitimacy of **surrogate mother** contracts. Mr. and Mrs. Stern entered into a surrogacy contract with Ms. Whitehead. She was impregnated with Mr. Stern's sperm and agreed to give up all parental rights in favor of the Sterns when the baby was born; Ms. Whitehead was to receive financial compensation in return. However, shortly after the birth she ran away with the child and refused to return it to the Sterns. The court held that surrogacy contracts involving financial payment were unenforceable and a violation of public policy, and that surrogate mothers have the right to change their minds after birth and assert their parental rights. In Baby M's situation, the courts held that the baby's "best interests" must be considered primary and awarded custody to Mr. Stern and visitation rights to Ms. Whitehead.

Beneficence: Action intended to benefit or promote the well-being of others. (*Benevolence* is the virtue or character trait by which one is disposed to act in a beneficent manner.) Historically, the ethics of Western Hippocratic medicine has been dominated by the twin professional obligations of beneficence and **nonmaleficence** ("do no harm"). While most persons accept some sense of obligation to exercise at least minimal beneficence toward others, many also hold themselves to obligations of *ideal* beneficence—that is, obligations to benefit others in ways not ordinarily accepted as morally obligatory within society, and based perhaps in a particular sense of altruism or religious conviction. In older terminology, acts of ideal beneficence are often described as **supererogatory** actions, meaning that which is above or beyond the call of moral duty or obligation. Some specific duties of benefi-cence, however, also arise within and because of particular moral relationships (e.g., parent, friend) or professional roles (e.g., physician, nurse, counselor, pastor). (See, for example, Tom L. Beauchamp and James F. Childress, *Principles of Biomedical Ethics*, 6th ed. [New York: Oxford University Press, 2009], especially chapter 6.)

Benign: Generally, having a nondangerous character that does not threaten health or life. A benign **tumor,** for instance, is one that is not cancerous, not **malignant**—that is, does not invade surrounding tissues or spread to other parts of the body.

Best interests: A legal (and moral) standard for **surrogate consent** to treatment or research participation on behalf of a now-incompetent individual who has never been compe-tent or who has never expressed any views or preferences that could guide the surrogate to a reliable **substituted judgment** for that individual in this situation. According to the best interests standard, the surrogate decision maker must protect the incompetent person's well-being by assessing the benefits and risks or inconveniences of all available options and then choosing that option that promises the greatest net benefit for the incompetent person. In many cases this will necessarily entail **"quality of life"** judgments by the surrogate on behalf of the incompetent person. When at least some general informa-tion about the incompetent person's values and desires can be known and applied to a weighing of predicted benefits or risks, then a *subjective* best interests standard may be applicable. When no such background knowledge is available, an *objective* best interest standard—based upon what benefits a reasonable person would likely seek, and what risks or discomforts a rea-sonable person would likely avoid—must be employed.

Bioengineering: (a) The application and integration of the principles of engineering and the natural sciences in the study of biology and physical and behavioral medicine. In its medical applications, bioengineering (also called biomedical engineering) is concerned with such pursuits as the development of new diagnostic imaging techniques, computer modeling of various organ functions, artificial organs and organ function replacement technologies, and new diagnostic instruments for blood analysis. (b) A synonym for **genetic engineering.**

Bioethics committee: See **institutional ethics committee**

Biological determinism: See **determinism**

Biometrics: The science and technology of authenticating a person's (or animal's) identity through measurement of that individual's physiological or behavioral features. Physiological biometrics identify individuals based on distinct anatomical or physiological traits. Applications would include, for example, iris or retina scans, fingerprint identification, vascular pattern analysis, and DNA analysis. Behavioral biometrics identify individuals based on measurement of distinct actions particular to that individual. Applications would include speech pattern recognition, signature analysis, and keystroke analysis.

Biotechnology: Scientific manipulation of living organisms, or parts of organisms, to make or modify products, to alter or improve plants or animals, or to develop microorganisms for specific uses. Examples include fermentation technologies to produce bread, cheese, beer, and so on; production of genetically modified organisms (GMOs) via **genetic engineering;** cloning technologies; stem cell research and therapies; and the production of antibiotics from organisms.

Blastocyst: A stage early in the development of the embryo, which consists of a sphere with an outer layer of cells, a fluid-filled cavity, and a inner cell mass of undifferentiated cells (the source of embryonic **stem cells**). The blastocyst will become a fetus if the blastocyst undergoes **implantation** (attachment) in the lining of a uterus. (See **embryonic development**)

Blastomere: A stage very early in the development of the embryo, which consists of a solid mass (**morula**) of same-size cells. (See **embryonic development**)

Brain death: Complete and irreversible cessation of brain function. The phrase is generally used to refer to *whole brain death*, which is the absence of all brain function as evidenced by profound coma, lack of spontaneous respiration, and absence of all brain stem reflexes. (*Upper brain death*, conversely, refers specifically to the irreversible loss of function of the cerebral cortex, which may leave brain stem reflexes, such as spontaneous respiration, intact.) Clinical diagnosis of what is now called (whole) brain death was first described in the medical literature in 1959 as "irreversible coma." (Another early term for this clinical phenomenon was "coma dépassé.) In 1968 an ad hoc committee of Harvard Medical School published a report describing the characteristics of "irreversible coma" as unreceptivity and unresponsivity, no movements or (unassisted) breathing, and no reflexes. A flat electroencephalogram (EEG) should provide corroboration of this diagnosis, and potentially reversible neurological conditions, such as those caused by hypothermia or barbiturate overdosage, must be ruled out. This set of clinical characteristics became known popularly as the Harvard criteria for irreversible coma. The President's Commission report on *Defining Death* (1981) recommended adoption and usage of similar diagnostic criteria and became the model for most state laws defining brain death. Also, the **Uniform Determination of Death Act (UDDA),** which is now part of statute law in most U.S. states, recognizes brain death (irreversible cessation of all functions of the entire brain, including the brain stem) along with circulatory-respiratory death (irreversible cessation of circulatory and respiratory functions) as legal "death." Yet because much of the original impetus to adopt "brain death" as a legal definition was based in the need to increase availability of cadaver organs for transplantation, some persons remain suspicious of the validity and application of this definition. And because a brain-dead but mechanically ventilated individual appears so "alive," some family members simply cannot accept that the individual is actually dead. Also, certain religious and cultural groups (e.g., Orthodox Judaism, and some Asian and Native American cultures) do not accept that death has occurred until all vital functions, including circulation and respiration, have ceased.

Buck v. Bell: A case argued before the U.S. Supreme Court (274 U.S. 200 [1927]) testing a Virginia law that allowed for the involuntary sterilization of certain mentally defective or otherwise "unfit" individuals for purposes of **eugenics.** Carrie Buck, the named plaintiff, was diagnosed as an epileptic, "feebleminded," and a "moral delinquent" because she had an illegitimate child. Her mother and her child were also described as "feebleminded." The lawsuit, brought in Ms. Buck's name, challenged the constitutionality of the 1924 Virginia Statute for Eugenical Sterilization. The Supreme Court majority found in favor of the State of Virginia (and, thus, other states that had similar laws). Justice Oliver Wendell Holmes's written opinion for the majority famously (or infamously) noted that "the principle that sustains compulsory vaccination is broad enough to cover cutting the Fallopian tubes. Three generations of imbeciles are enough." (See, for example, Paul A. Lombardo, *Three Generations, No Imbeciles: Eugenics, the Supreme Court, and Buck v. Bell* [Baltimore: Johns Hopkins University Press, 2008].)

ↄ C ↄ

Canterbury v. Spence: A court case heard by the U.S. Court of Appeals for the District of Columbia Circuit (464 F.2D 762 [D.C. CIR. 1972]) regarding standards for disclosure of risks in **informed consent** for treatment. The plaintiff had undergone surgery for a ruptured disk in his back and then developed urinary incontinence and some paralysis after a postsurgical fall. He claimed that he had never been warned of the possibility of paralysis as a risk of the surgery when consent had been given. The court held that a physician must not simply follow customs of the profession in disclosing information prior to treatment but must instead apply a "patient-centered" standard of disclosure that provides the patient with all information "material" to his making an "intelligent choice." Thus, "all risks potentially affecting the decision must be unmasked."

Capacity, decisional: See **decisional capacity**

Cardioversion: The restoration of a normal heart rhythm in cases of too-rapid heartbeat or cardiac arrhythmias (irregular, ineffective contractions of the heart muscle). One form of cardioversion is accomplished via electric shock (electric cardioversion) using a defibrillator with electrode paddles placed externally on the chest to pass electrical current through the heart, "converting" the abnormal cardiac electrical impulses to a normal cardiac rhythm. In some cases an internal cardiac defibrillator is implanted under the skin to provide electric shock when abnormal heart rhythm develops. The other main form of cardioversion is pharmacologic cardioversion, in which drugs are used to restore a more normal heart rhythm.

Care, ethics of: A group or family of approaches to moral reasoning that emphasize the nature and quality of significant relationships and the care, commitment, and willingness to act on the other's behalf that characterize those relationships. The ethics of care has emerged largely from feminist ethical analysis. An early example was the work of psychologist Carol Gilligan in *In a Different Voice: Psychological Theory and Women's Development* (Cambridge, MA: Harvard University Press, 1982). Gilligan held that women's moral development is different from men's, and that women tend to think morally from what she calls an "ethic of care," a relationality and responsivity model, while men tend to think morally from an "ethic of rights and justice" characterized by dispassionate analysis and adjudication of impartial moral principles. Interpretations of an ethics of care have also been prominent in the literature of the nursing profession, offering understandings of the particular form of "caring" necessary in the relationship between nurses and those in their care. One of the earliest sustained developments of an ethics of care and its implications was Nel Noddings' *Caring: A Feminine Approach to Ethics and Moral Education* (Berkeley: University of California Press, 1984).

Casuistry: Essentially, argument by cases (from Latin *casus,* meaning case). In some older definitions the term referred to the application of general ethical principles in the resolution of moral conflicts or dilemmas. In contemporary applied ethics it refers to that approach in moral reasoning wherein one tries to determine the correct moral conclusion in a particular case (involving a moral problem or dilemma) by drawing parallels between that case and other "paradigms" or "pure cases" for which the correct moral conclusion has already been agreed upon. This form of reasoning has been the foundation of Anglo-American common law, in which new cases are adjudicated based on their relevant similarity to previous cases in which a judgment (precedent) has been established. (See, for example, Albert Jonsen and Stephen Toulmin, *The Abuse of Casuistry: A History of Moral Reasoning* [Berkeley: University of California Press, 1988].)

Categorical imperative: In the deontological moral theory of Immanuel Kant, the supreme moral principle from which all duties and obligations can be derived. (See **deontology**)

Cell nucleus: See **nucleus, cell**

Chorionic villus sampling (CVS):   A **prenatal diagnosis** technique in which a small sample of tissue (chorionic villi) from the placenta is obtained and analyzed to detect genetic and chromosomal abnormalities in the fetus. CVS is usually performed at ten to twelve weeks of pregnancy (as measured from the woman's last menstrual period). The tissue sample is obtained using an ultrasound-guided thin tube (through the cervix) or needle (through the abdomen). CVS is not employed as often as **amniocentesis,** the most widely used technique for prenatal diagnosis, and it entails a risk of miscarriage somewhat higher than that with amniocentesis. However, it can be performed at a relatively earlier stage in a pregnancy. It is often recommended when the pregnant woman is age 35 or older (and thus at increased risk of bearing a child with certain chromosomal defects), when a genetic or chromosomal abnormality has been diagnosed in a previous pregnancy, or when a family medical history indicates an increased risk of bearing a child with a significant genetic disorder.

Chromosomes: Threadlike structures within the **nucleus** of a cell, composed of very long **DNA** molecules (with specialized associated proteins) and carrying most of the hereditary information of the organism. The functional units of DNA, which together form a chromosome, are **genes,** each of which contains the genetic code or instructions for making a specific protein. Normal human body (somatic) cell nuclei contain forty-six chromosomes in twenty-three matched pairs, whereas normal human reproductive (gamete) cell nuclei contain a single set of twenty-three chromosomes.

Clinical trial: A form of medical **experimentation** in which investigators manipulate the administration of some new drug or other treatment and measure the effect(s) of that manipulation. The best-known form of clinical trial is the **randomized clinical trial,** or RCT, in which subjects are randomly chosen to receive the new form of therapy under study, or an inactive **placebo** (in "placebo control" trials), or the current standard-of-care therapy (in an "active control" trial). Careful measurements are then taken of the relative effects of the different forms of therapy (or placebo) to determine their relative therapeutic value. RCTs are "single-blind" (in which the subjects have no knowledge of, or in some cases no choice about, which form of therapy or placebo they are selected to receive) or "double-blind" (in which neither the investigators nor the subjects know, or choose, which subjects are receiving which treatment option). In the United States, the Food and Drug Administration (FDA) requires evidence from clinical trials of the effectiveness and relative safety of all new drugs and other medical therapies prior to their approval for marketing. For pharmaceuticals, the drug-development process usually proceeds through four stages, or phases, of clinical trials over many years. Phase I trials are the first human testing of the new therapy and usually involve administering it to small groups of healthy human volunteers to gauge its toxicity, tolerability, pharmacodynamics, and pharmacokinetics. This is a form of "nontherapeutic" research because the subjects have no clinical need for the therapy being tested. (Because of their high levels of toxicity, some phase I trials of new cancer and HIV drugs are conducted using volunteers who are sick and in the last stages of those diseases.) Phase II trials involve larger groups of subjects—in this case, persons who are sick with a condition for which the new treatment might be useful—to assess the clinical efficacy of the therapy. (Many new drugs fail during phase II trials as poor efficacy or toxic side effects are discovered.) Phase II and successive phases are forms of "therapeutic research" inasmuch as the treatment under study may have therapeutic benefit for the particular subject. Phase III trials involve large groups of patient-subjects and are designed to assess definitively the new therapy's clinical efficacy, especially in comparison to other therapeutic alternatives currently available. Phase IV trials are conducted after the new therapy has been marketed and involve safety surveillance and ongoing technical refinement of the therapy. These long-term trials may discover other applications and other long-term side effects of the therapy that were not revealed in phases I–III due to the limited populations and time periods in those phases.

Cloning: The production of a *clone* (broadly, a genetic replica of a **DNA** molecule, cell, tissue, organ, or entire animal or plant; or, more specifically, an organism with the same nuclear **genome** of another organism). For humans and other animals, cloning involves generating an individual whose nuclear **genes** are derived from a **diploid** cell of another embryo, fetus, or already-born person of the same species. The best-known and most successful cloning technology to date is somatic cell nuclear transfer (SCNT), in which the

nucleus from a somatic (nonreproductive) cell of an individual is transferred into an unfertilized **ovum** (egg cell) whose nucleus (containing the maternal **chromosomes**) has been removed; the ovum is then stimulated to begin dividing, leading to the development of a new organism with the same chromosomal complement (genome) as the individual from whom the somatic cell nucleus was taken. Cloning technology may be employed for both reproductive and nonreproductive purposes. Reproductive cloning includes implantation of the resulting (cloned) organism into a woman's uterus with the goal of pregnancy and childbirth. The first reported successful reproductive cloning of a mammal via SCNT was a sheep, known to the world as **"Dolly,"** born in 1996. Nonreproductive or therapeutic cloning is undertaken to produce early embryos whose **stem cells** can be harvested for medical research and therapeutic purposes. (See related entries at **embryo splitting** and **parthenogenesis.**)

Coma (From Greek *koma* = deep sleep):   A profound state of unconsciousness from which one cannot be awakened and in which one does not respond normally to light or pain, does not make voluntary actions, and does not exhibit sleep–wake cycles. Unlike sleep, coma is not always reversible; unlike stupor, coma is characterized by lack of suitable response to all verbal or noxious stimuli; unlike **persistent vegetative state (PVS),** coma is characterized by no sleep–wake cycles, spontaneous movements, eye-opening, or response to external stimuli. The most common causes of comas are brain trauma (from pressure, **hypoxia,** altered pH, chemical or nutrient imbalance, drug intoxication, infection, and so on), malignant **neoplasm,** or focal lesion or stroke. Usually, a coma will last for only a few days to a few weeks, and rarely beyond two to four weeks. Comas generally resolve into recovery or progress into a persistent vegetative state.

Communitarianism: In contemporary philosophy, a theory emphasizing the influence of society in defining and shaping individuals (as opposed to liberalism's emphasis on individual choice as the foundational basis for society) and emphasizing the traditions, practices and histories of communities as the source of one's beliefs and values (as opposed to liberalism's emphasis on reason's recognition of abstract principles and values). Although the term "communitarian" dates from the mid-nineteenth century, modern communitarianism has emerged largely as a critique of liberal theories of justice (notably John Rawls' influential *A Theory of Justice* [Cambridge, MA: Harvard University Press, 1971]). Among the "liberal" assumptions most criticized by communitiarians are the centrality of individual **autonomy,** the primacy of personal rights held against the state, and the idea that governments should remain neutral toward competing values and conceptions of the good life within society. (See, e.g., Michael Sandel, *Liberalism and the Limits of Justice* [Cambridge, MA: Cambridge University Press, 1982].)

Competence: Generally, the mental or volitional ability necessary to perform some particular task. Because any competence is relative to a specific task, the criteria for judging or assessing competence will be relative to those abilities necessary to perform the task in question. Legally, competence can refer to a judicial or other legal recognition that an individual possesses the necessary rational and volitional abilities to, for example, understand legal charges and participate in a criminal trial, execute a valid will, decide about one's financial affairs, or give valid consent to medical treatment or research participation. In health care settings, the term "competence" is often used to refer to the more specific matter of **decisional capacity**—that is, an individual's ability to make health care decisions for her own reasons and in her own best interests.

(See, e.g., Bernard Gert, Charles M. Culver, and K. Danner Clouser, *Bioethics: A Return to Fundamentals* [New York: Oxford University Press, 1997], especially chapter 6.)

Conceptus: A term used to describe the products of fertilization or conception: the embryo and the embryonic part of the placenta and other associated membranes. (See **embryonic development**)

Confidentiality: The practice (and the moral duty) of not disclosing to third parties information received in confidence from another person without the consent of that person. Rules of confidentiality in clinical practice have long been recognized in codes of medical ethics, including the Hippocratic oath. While professional commitments to honor patient confidentiality in health care have generally been respected in law as well (at least in Western societies), exceptions have been recognized in which the maintenance of confidentiality might lead to a threat of harm to third parties. For example, the majority opinion of the California Supreme Court in the **Tarasoff case** (1976) held that the confidentiality of patient–psychotherapist communications must yield to the duty of disclosure when necessary to avert danger to others threatened by that patient.

Conflict of interest: A situation in which an individual (or group) is subject to influences that have a significant potential to lead him (or them) to act contrary to his (or their) professional or ethical responsibility. In business, for example, conflicts of interest arise when persons in positions of trust are led by self-interest to conduct their entrusted activities in ways that may not be in the company's or client's best interests. In health care a conflict of interest may arise, for example, when a physician considers stopping a patient's treatment with a known effective drug to begin treatment with a new drug being marketed by a company in which that physician owns stock.

Conjoined twins (or Siamese twins):   Monozygotic twins whose bodies are joined together at birth. (See **twins**)

Consequentialism: A term applied to theories of moral justification which state that the moral rightness or wrongness of any act must be judged solely in terms of the goodness or badness of that act's predicted consequences. The best-known form of consequentialism is **utilitarianism,** which holds that one must always act so as to produce the greatest utility—that is, the greatest good and least bad consequences for the maximal number of all those affected. *Ethical egoism* holds that moral right, wrong, and obligation depend upon the predicted consequences for the individual moral agent alone. *Altruism* holds that moral right, wrong, and obligation depend upon the predicted consequences for everyone other than the moral agent.

Cruzan case: 1990 U.S. Supreme Court case (*Cruzan v. Director, Missouri Department of Health,* 497 U.S. 261 [1990]) that addressed withdrawal of life support (in this case, artificial nutrition and hydration) for incompetent persons. Nancy Cruzan had been in a **persistent vegetative state (PVS)** for more than four years when her parents concluded that she would not wish to be maintained in that condition and sued for permission to have her artificial nutrition and hydration discontinued. The local court granted their request, but that decision was overturned by the Missouri Supreme Court, which held that the family had not produced "clear and convincing evidence" that she would wish to die under such circumstances and upheld a Missouri law that proscribed the removal of feeding and hydration under any circumstances. The U.S. Supreme Court held that all competent adult persons have the constitutional right to accept or reject medical treatment, even life-preserving treatment, and that this right does not end when one becomes incompetent. However, the court also held that the individual states are free to determine the requisite standard of proof regarding the previously expressed wishes of a now-incompetent person. And because Missouri's required standard of "clear and convincing evidence" of Nancy Cruzan's own previously expressed wish not to be kept alive in a persistent vegetative state had not been met, the Cruzan family's claim on her behalf was not granted. Thereafter, the Cruzan family filed their legal suit once again at the local level, and the same judge who had heard the initial case determined that they had provided "clear and convincing evidence" of Nancy's wishes. Her artificial nutrition and hydration were discontinued, and she died on December 26, 1990.

CVS: See **chorionic villus sampling**

Cyclosporine: See **transplantation, organ and tissue**

D

D&C (dilation and curettage): A surgical procedure involving dilation of the cervix followed by scraping or suctioning of the lining of the uterus. D&C is used in some cases to procure **abortion.** (See **abortion**)

D&E (dilation and evacuation): Surgical procedure involving dilation of the cervix followed by removal of fetus and placenta via surgical instruments or vacuum suction, or both. (See **abortion**)

D&X (dilation and extraction): Surgical procedure involving cervical dilation followed by partial delivery of the intact fetus feet first; then a sharp instrument is inserted into the back of the fetus's head and the brain is suctioned before delivery is completed. (See **abortion**)

DBS: See **deep brain stimulation**

DCD: See **donation after cardiac death**

Dead donor rule: The moral and legal requirements that transplantable vital organs may not be removed from a potential cadaver organ donor until after that individual is determined to be clinically dead (according to criteria for whole **brain death** or due to "irreversible cessation of circulatory and respiratory functions") and that the removal of organs cannot be the cause of death. There has been much controversy over whether the dead donor rule might be "relaxed" to allow for harvesting organs from persons who have not experienced *whole* brain death but merely *upper* (cerebral) brain death, and whether a category of allowable donors should be established for those born without a functioning upper brain (i.e., babies with **the neural tube defect** anencephaly). (See also **donation after cardiac death**)

Decisional capacity: The ability to make health care (or other) decisions for oneself, weighing information received along with one's needs, goals, and interests, and reaching conclusions that reflect one's values and best interests. Decisional capacity may be compromised by temporary causes such as sedation, hypoxia, physical or mental stress, and alcohol or chemical intoxication or by longer-term causes such as memory loss and dementia. As with the more general legal notion of **competence,** assessments of decisional capacity are task specific, and even context specific. One's capacity to reflect upon and reach conclusions regarding one kind of decision does not necessarily imply similar capacity or incapacity for other forms of decision making.

Deep brain stimulation (DBS):   A neurosurgical procedure in which a device called a "brain pacemaker" is surgically implanted to send electrical impulses to particular areas of the brain. It has been effective in the treatment of essential tremor, Parkinson's disease, some forms of clinical depression, and dystonia (a neurological disorder in which involuntary muscle contractions cause abnormal postures or repetitive and twisting movements).

Delayed animation: Belief that the human embryo/fetus takes on human form—that is, becomes "animated" or "ensouled"—at some point in development after conception. (See **animation**)

Deontology: Generally, a theory of moral obligation that claims that the rightness or wrongness of human actions must be determined with reference to characteristics of those actions other than simply the goodness or badness of their predicted consequences. In this sense, deontology has been seen as a theoretical counterpoint to **consequentialism** and **utilitarianism.** One very ancient form of deontology, divine command theory, holds that moral rightness and wrongness can be identified and measured only by the will of the divine (and that the divine will has been sufficiently revealed to human consciousness to make correct moral choice possible, through obedience to divine command). Another well-known deontology, that of Immanuel Kant, holds that all moral obligations can be derived from a single ultimate moral norm, the "categorical imperative." Of Kant's several expressions of the categorical imperative, his first was "act only according to that maxim by which you can at the same time will that it should become a universal law." His second formulation, often cited in discussions of the ethics of medical experimentation, was that one must "act so that you treat humanity . . . always as an end and never as a means only." Kant believed that we should always act not only in accordance with but also for the sake of rationally perceived moral obligation, and that our particular moral obligations are defined by moral rules that are in turn derived from the categorical imperative. (See Immanuel Kant, *Groundwork of the Metaphysic of Morals,* trans. H. J. Paton [New York: Harper and Row, 1964].) One other notable form of deontology is that of the twentieth-century British philosopher W. D. Ross, who claimed that our recognition of basic moral obligations emerges from our experience of various social structures and relationships. Furthermore, in contrast to Kant, Ross held that these obligations are fundamentally plural rather than emerging from a single categorical imperative, and that they can and do conflict with one another in a variety of circumstances. Thus, he claimed, we must understand these basic moral obligations not as absolute duties but rather as prima facie duties—that is, as obligations generally to be fulfilled but which may need to be overridden by another stronger or more pressing prima facie duty in situations of conflict of duties. (See W. D. Ross, *The Right and the Good* [Oxford: Clarendon Press, 1930].) Most deontological theories, including those of Kant and Ross, take the form of "rule deontology," meaning that our fundamental moral obligations are expressed in moral rules that are consistently applicable. A much rarer form, "act deontology," would hold that our moral obligations must somehow be discerned in the moment of moral choice—an approach in which consistency, predictability, and rational analysis of moral choice would be difficult at best.

Deoxyribonucleic acid (DNA):   A chemical (a nucleic acid) that usually exists in the form of a long, twisted ladder-like shape (a double helix) and contains the genetic instructions that direct the development of all cellular life forms (and most viruses). DNA is composed of a pair of molecules, each of which consists of a long chain of chemical nucleotides: adenine (A), thymine (T), cytosine (C), and guanine (G). The two chains are held together with hydrogen bonds between nucleotide "pairs," A–T (or T–A) and C–G (or G–C). At cell division the two strands of DNA (in the nucleus of the cell) split apart (or "unzip"), and each becomes a template for the formation of a new strand that will have the same A–T, T–A, G–C, and C–G pairings. The sequence of these base pairs will determine the genetic information passed along to offspring of the organism. In human beings, most DNA is found in the cell nucleus; however, some DNA is also present outside the nucleus in organelles called **mitochondria. Genes** are segments of DNA strands that encode for the production of particular proteins. **Chromosomes** contain long chain-like collections of genes. The entire DNA complement of an organism is known as its **genome.** In human beings each **somatic** cell is **diploid,** that is, it contains twenty-three pairs of chromosomes, one chromosome in each pair from the father and one from the mother (plus some mitochondrial DNA from the mother's egg cell). **Germ cells** (ovum and sperm), however, are **haploid,** containing only twenty-three chromosomes (half of each paired set of chromosomes from each parent).

Descriptive ethics: A form of ethical analysis that involves a factual examination of the moral behavior and belief of persons or groups, much like the social sciences. It does not seek to answer moral questions about what ought to be done or judged; rather, it seeks empirical knowledge about what is believed and acted upon in the moral lives of persons as well as what causal factors may explain why those moral views are held. (See **ethics**)

Determinism: In philosophical terms, the notion that all events, including human thoughts and actions, are effects caused by a constant chain of prior events or occurrences, with no genuinely random events and no true freedom of the will. **Genetic determinism** refers to the idea that certain physical and behavioral traits are expressions of, and thus are necessarily determined by, the presence of particular genes or groups of genes in that individual's cells.

Dialysis, renal: A form of artificial replacement for lost kidney function, used in persons who have experienced sudden but potentially reversible loss of kidney function (acute renal failure) or permanent loss of kidney function (end-stage renal failure). Normal kidneys remove from the bloodstream both excess fluid and the body's chemical waste products (e.g., urea and excess potassium). Renal dialysis must replace both of these removal functions. Dialysis operates by causing the diffusion of certain chemical solutes through a semipermeable membrane. In *hemodialysis* a patient's blood runs through tubing into a machine and into contact with a semipermeable membrane with dialysis fluid on its other side, so that blood solutes and excess fluid are caused to diffuse into the dialysis fluid. In *peritoneal dialysis* the membrane of the patient's own peritoneum (the sac surrounding the intestines) serves as the semipermeable membrane for dialysis. Fluid in various osmotic strengths is introduced into the peritoneal sac and is left there for a period of time so that solutes and excess bodily fluid can pass across the peritoneal membrane into the fluid, which is then drained out of the body. Another form of treatment similar to hemodialysis is *hemofiltration*, which uses a more porous semipermeable membrane and artificially replaces desired solutes and fluid volume after large quantities of fluid and solutes have passed through the membrane.

Dilation and curettage (D&C):   See **abortion; D&C**

Dilation and evacuation (D&E):   See **abortion; D&E**

Dilation and extraction (D&X):   See **abortion; D&X**

Diploid: The term used to describe a cell that contains two copies (homologues) of each chromosome, generally with one set of copies from the mother and one from the father. In human beings, virtually every **somatic cell** (body cell) is diploid, containing the full diploid complement of forty-six (twenty-three times two) chromosomes. (See also **haploid**)

Disorder, genetic: See **genetic disorder**

Divine command theory: A theory of moral obligation holding that moral rightness and wrongness can be identified and measured only by the will of the divine (and that the divine will has been sufficiently revealed to human consciousness to make correct moral choice possible, through obedience to divine command). (See **deontology**)

Dizygotic twin: One of a pair of individuals developing together in a uterus but from two separate fertilized **zygotes.** Dizygotic twins are often referred to as "fraternal twins." (See **twins**)

DNA: See **deoxyribonucleic acid**

DNA databanks: Collections of DNA sequencing data that provide genetic identification of particular individuals. The U.S. military, for example, maintains a databank of identifying DNA profiles for all its members, and all fifty U.S. states maintain databanks of DNA profiles of those convicted of crimes. (See **DNA fingerprinting**)

DNA fingerprinting (or DNA profiling, or genetic fingerprinting): The process of distinguishing one individual within a species from others in that species through examination of DNA samples from blood, semen, saliva, and other body tissues and fluids. The practice was first introduced in the United Kingdom in 1985. While most individuals within a species will have the vast majority of their DNA in common, DNA fingerprinting seeks to identify numbers of certain variable repeating sequences of DNA at particular chromosomal loci. Because of the very high probability that these sequences at a given locus will differ between unrelated individuals, multiple sequences at multiple loci are identified to establish near-certain statistical probability that a given DNA sample must have come from only one particular individual (unless that individual has an identical twin, who would share the same DNA sequencing). Thus this form of identification has been used widely in forensic science. The first conviction of a crime based on analysis of a DNA sample left at the crime scene occurred in 1987; the first exoneration of a convicted felon based on evidence from DNA fingerprinting occurred in 1989. Vast **DNA databanks** of identifying information from DNA fingerprinting have been established in many industrial nations, and all fifty U.S. states hold banks of DNA profiles. In addition to its forensic applications, DNA fingerprinting has been used to provide a more precise means of identification for military personnel in case of battlefield casualty, to identify dead bodies, to prove or disprove paternity, and to trace lines of ancestry (based upon familial DNA sequencing patterns). Due to concerns about privacy and the control of personal identifying information, there has been much controversy about the circumstances in which DNA sampling legitimately may be mandated and about who controls or has access to the banked DNA information.

DNA sequence. See **deoxyribonucleic acid**

DNR (do not resuscitate):   A medical order, usually in written form and signed by a physician, stating that resuscitation efforts should not be attempted for a particular person if she experiences cardiac (heart) or pulmonary (lung) arrest. Ideally, a DNR order should be sought by the person who does not wish to be subjected to resuscitative interventions. Some DNR requests are incorporated in a person's **advance directive** for health care; others may be sought on behalf of an incompetent or never-competent person by her legal guardian, surrogate, or health care proxy.

"Dolly:" The name given to a female sheep born in 1996 at the Roslin Institute in Scotland. She was the first mammal born after successful cloning via the somatic cell nuclear transfer procedure. The nuclear DNA from which Dolly developed was taken from the mammary cell of a six-year-old ewe. Dolly lived for six years.

Dominant gene: See **disorder, genetic**

Donation after cardiac death (DCD): A policy regarding the retrieval of organs or tissues for transplantation from deceased persons. Since the 1960s, cadaver organ-retrieval policies have generally required that potential donors meet the criteria for whole **brain death** before organs may be removed. This not only ensured that the donor was indeed clinically dead before vital organs were removed but it also allowed for adequate perfusion of transplantable organs with oxygenated blood (necessary for their vitality) up until their removal from the donor body (whose heartbeat and respiration are maintained mechanically). In contrast, DCD policies allow for a procedure in which some dying (not brain-dead) persons may be allowed to experience cessation of heartbeat and respiration after removal of life-support technology. Then transplantable organs or tissues are immediately removed, or the donor is connected to machinery that perfuses the body with oxygenated blood mechanically (without heartbeat) until organs or tissues may be surgically removed for transplant purposes. Early (and some current) DCD policies refer to these donors as "non–heart-beating donors" (NHBD). One of the earliest and most widely discussed policies for NHBD organ retrievals was developed in the early 1990s at the University of Pittsburgh hospitals and became known as the Pittsburgh Protocol. Later, the Institute of Medicine examined a variety of NHBD protocols and offered recommendations for their clarification and standardization. (See Institute of Medicine, *Non-Heart-Beating Organ Transplantation: Medical and Ethical Issues in Procurement* [Washington, DC: National Academies Press, 1997]; and Institute of Medicine, *Non-Heart-Beating Organ Transplantation: Practice and Protocols* [Washington, DC: National Academies Press, 2000].)

Do no harm: See **nonmaleficence; primum non nocere**

Double effect, rule or principle of: A guide for moral reasoning developed in Catholic moral theology often attributed to Thomas Aquinas. (See, e.g., Aquinas's discussion of the morality of killing in self-defense in his *Summa Theologiae* II–II, q.64, art.7.) It seeks to explain those circumstances in which it is morally acceptable to perform an action that will predictably lead to a desired good consequence or effect even though it will also predictably result in an evil consequence or effect (hence the designation "double effect"). Four conditions are generally applied to justify such an action. First, the action itself must be morally good or at least morally neutral (i.e., not intrinsically evil). Second, only the good effect may be morally intended, even though the evil effect may be foreseen. Third, the intended good effect must result directly from the action in question; it must not result from the (unintended) evil effect. In other words, the evil effect must not be directly produced to then yield the good effect. And, fourth, there must be proportionality between the good and evil effects—that is, the evil must be outweighed by the good in the predicted outcome. Examples of traditional applications of the rule of double effect would include the justification of "collateral damage" to innocent civilians in wartime (when such casualties are the proportionate and foreseen but unintended results of attacks on morally legitimate military targets) and the use of large doses of narcotic sedatives for the treatment of otherwise untreatable pain in terminal illness (even though such dosages may have the foreseen but unintended consequence of suppressing respiration and thus leading to an earlier death for the patient). Since 1895 the Roman Catholic Church has recognized two instances of surgically induced "justified fetal death" that are not considered **abortion** due to the rule of double effect: cases involving ectopic pregnancy or cancerous uterus. In both of these circumstances, fetal death results as a by-product of the surgical removal of an organ with a pathologic condition in order to save the woman's life (i.e., a fallopian tube that would eventually rupture as the fetus develops, leading to potentially fatal hemorrhage; or removal of a uterus containing not only a fetus but also a fast-growing cancer that would eventually kill mother and fetus). In recent decades some Catholic moral theologians have suggested that the real heart of the double effect doctrine lies not so much in the question of whether the good and evil effects are directly or indirectly intended but rather in the question of proportionality between the good and evil effects (and thus "proportionate reason" for the action in question). (See, e.g., R. A. McCormick and P. Ramsey, eds., *Doing Evil to Achieve Good: Moral Choice in Conflict Situations* [Chicago: Loyola University Press, 1978].)

Double helix: The helical, ladder-like structure of the DNA molecule (see **deoxyribonucleic acid**).

Down syndrome (Trisomy 21):   See **aneuploidy**

Durable power of attorney for health care (DPoA):   A document by which an individual may designate a particular person or persons to act as his health care proxy for treatment choices, in the event that he becomes incapable of forming or expressing those choices in the future. In other words, a durable power of attorney document represents the author's prospective consent to those forms of treatment chosen on his behalf by the designated proxy or advocate. (See also **advance directive**)

Duty to warn: The moral and legal (in tort law) obligation of one party, who is aware of a significant hazard or threat of harm to a second party, to warn that second party of the existence of the threat or hazard. Product liability lawsuits often involve a manufacturer's failure to fulfill its duty to warn in cases in which its products pose some risk of harm, which is known to the manufacturer, to consumers who are unaware of that risk. In the well-known **Tarasoff case** (*Tarasoff v. Regents of the University of California*) in 1976, the majority opinion of the California Supreme Court established a strong duty to warn on the part of mental health therapists. While the Tarasoff case applied only to California jurisdictions, all fifty U.S. states have adopted, via legal precedents or statute law, some version of the duty to warn established in that case. (See **Tarasoff case**)

ECLS (extracorporeal life support):   See **extracorporeal membrane oxygenation**

ECMO: See **extracorporeal membrane oxygenation**

ECT: See **electroconvulsive therapy**

Ectogenesis: The process of embryonic and fetal development outside the womb. In humans, this would require the development of an "artificial womb" to support fetal development. While ectogenesis is not possible at this time, researchers have been able to produce implantation of an embryo in laboratory-grown uterine tissue, and have created artificial amniotic fluid for the support of very premature infants.

Ectopic pregnancy: A pregnancy in which the fertilized ovum implants and develops in tissue other than the uterine wall. In humans, most ectopic pregnancies occur with implantation in the fallopian tube (hence the common term "tubal pregnancy"), but ectopic pregnancy involving cervical, ovarian, or abdominal implantation is also possible. Since 1895, ectopic pregnancy (particularly fallopian tube pregnancy) has been identified by the Roman Catholic Church as one of only two clinical indications for surgical intervention (in this case, removal of the involved fallopian tube) that will predictably cause fetal death, based upon reasoning summarized in the **double effect** principle.

Egg donation: See **gamete donation**

Electroconvulsive therapy (ECT):   A psychiatric treatment procedure in which electrical current is passed through the brain to induce a bilateral clonic seizure, characterized by convulsions and unconsciousness for at least sixty seconds. It is not understood exactly how ECT affects an individual's mental state or condition. The procedure was introduced in the 1930s as a treatment for schizophrenia, and its use was later broadened to include a variety of other diagnosed conditions. Its use diminished in the late twentieth century as more effective drug therapies became available. Contemporary use of ECT is generally reserved for cases of bipolar disorder and chronic depression in which other forms of therapy have not produced positive results. Early ECT treatments were performed without anesthesia and often resulted in broken bones and other injuries from the induced seizures; modern ECT treatments include the use of anesthesia and muscle relaxants. Because of ECT's history of overuse for some conditions, its abuse as a form of punishment for some patients, and uncertainty about its long-term effects, it remains a very controversial form of therapy.

Eleemosynary health care institutions: Hospitals, clinics, and other health care institutions that operate on a nonprofit basis and provide some degree of uncompensated or "charity" care.

ELSI: The ethical, legal, and social issues research program, which was instituted as part of the **Human Genome Project (HGP).** The various investigational and educational projects encompassed by ELSI became the largest bioethics program in the world, enabled in large part by funding amounting to

3 to 5 percent of the annual Human Genome Project budgets of the U.S. National Institutes of Health and the Department of Energy.

Emancipated minor: A child under the age of majority (eighteen years in the United States) who has been granted the status of adulthood for purposes of marriage, financial independence, or medical decision making by court order or other formal legal arrangement.

Embryo: See **embryonic development**

Embryo adoption: The transfer of a fertilized embryo, conceived through **in vitro fertilization,** to the uterus of a female who desires to "adopt" the embryo and bring it to birth. This procedure is usually sought by persons who wish to prevent the biological parents' donation of the embryo for embryonic **stem cell** research or other embryonic research.

Embryo donation: A form of **embryo transfer** in which the genetic parents (who provide the egg and sperm for in vitro fertilization) authorize transfer of the early embryo to the uterus of another female for implantation and pregnancy.

Embryo lavage: An alternative form of **embryo donation** in which an early embryo is washed out of a woman's reproductive tract and transferred to another woman's uterus for implantation and pregnancy. In this procedure, a fertile female egg donor is artificially inseminated, then one or more fertilized early embryos are lavaged (washed) from her reproductive tract and transferred via catheter into the uterus of another woman, hormonally prepared for implantation of the embryo, who wishes to become pregnant.

Embryo splitting: A term used to describe a process of artificial twinning in which one or more cells from the early embryo are separated from it and caused to begin their own independent processes of cell division and multiplication, leading to identical **twins,** triplets, quadruplets, and so on.

Embryo transfer: A step in the process of **in vitro fertilization** (a form of **assisted reproductive technology**) in which one or more fertilized early embryos (three to six days after fertilization) are transferred via a catheter into the uterus of a woman with the intention of establishing a pregnancy. Ethical questions have been voiced as to the nonnatural character of pregnancy resulting from this procedure. Other ethical concerns have been raised about the number of embryos to be transferred in the procedure. While the transfer of multiple embryos increases the prospect that at least one of them will implant in the uterine wall and establish pregnancy, it also increases the risk of multiple pregnancies beyond the number desired by the parents or even beyond the normal uterine capacity for sustaining pregnancy to birth.

Embryogenesis: The process of formation and development of the embryo. (See **embryonic development**)

Embryonic development: In human biology, the development of the organism (embryo) from the point of conception or **fertilization** (the joining of egg and sperm cells to begin a new and genetically unique organism) until the end of the eighth week, at which point the embryo is identified as a **fetus.** This process begins with the **zygote,** the one-cell product of fertilization. Multiple cell divisions then occur, eventually creating a solid mass (**morula**) of same-size cells called blastomeres. Then, about five days after fertilization, these cells form a blastocyst, a sphere with an outer layer of cells, a fluid-filled cavity, and an inner cell mass of undifferentiated cells (the source of embryonic **stem cells**) that will become the fetus if the blastocyst undergoes **implantation** (attachment) in the lining of a uterus. In humans, implantation occurs seven to fourteen days after fertilization. As the blastocyst undergoes further development of differentiated cell types and inner and outer cell layers, it is known as a gastrula. Eventually, interior passages and organs will develop, a process called organogenesis. At the end of the eighth week of development, the human embryo has rudimentary limbs, toes, and fingers, measures 0.8–1.2 inches in length, weighs 0.04–0.16 ounces, and has early forms of major organ systems. From that point until birth, it is known as a fetus.

Embryonic germ cells (EG):   Cells that originate from the primordial reproductive cells of the developing fetus and that have regenerative properties similar to those of embryonic **stem cells.**

Embryonic stem cells (ES):   See **stem cells**

Emergency Medical Treatment and Active Labor Act (EMTALA): Passed by the U.S. Congress in 1986, the EMTALA requires hospital emergency rooms and other emergency service providers to treat persons in active labor or with life-threatening conditions regardless of their ability to pay, their citizenship, or their legal status. The act applies to all health care facilities and emergency medical services receiving federal funds. It mandates that patients who are uninsured or unable to pay for care may not be transferred to another institution until their condition is stabilized or unless their condition requires treatment elsewhere. EMTALA was passed in the wake of news reports concerning persons with life-threatening conditions who died after being rejected by hospital emergency rooms because they were unable to pay for treatment.

Encephalitis: Inflammation of the brain.

Encephalocele: A **neural tube defect** in which one or more plates in the developing skull fail to seal, so that brain tissue and its membrane covering protrude through the gap in the skull. (See **neural tube defect**)

Encephalopathy: Any degenerative disease of the brain.

End: In moral reasoning, the aim, goal, purpose, or intended outcome of a particular choice or action. (See **means and ends**)

Ensoulment: See **animation**

Enzyme: A large chemical molecule, usually a protein, that catalyzes (enables and speeds up) a particular chemical reaction. Enzymes are essential to sustaining biological processes, and many human diseases are the result of enzyme deficiencies. For example, phenylketonuria (PKU), an inborn error of metabolism, is caused by a mutation of the enzyme phenylalanine hydroxylase. As a result, the body cannot convert the amino acid phenylalanine into tyrosine, and the resulting buildup of phenylalanine may lead to mental retardation and neurological and other problems unless the dietary intake of phenylalanine is strictly controlled.

Equipoise: In medical **experimentation,** the state of genuine uncertainty about which treatment "arm" in a **randomized clinical trial** may actually provide the safest and most effective form of treatment for human subjects enrolled in the trial. As an ethical requirement, equipoise means that a subject should never be enrolled in a randomized clinical trial unless there is substantial uncertainty about which form of treatment being tested would provide the greatest benefit for that subject. It is based in the moral principles of **beneficence** and **nonmaleficence**—that the physician-researcher's primary obligation is always to provide the greatest known benefit and avoid the most known harms for each patient-subject, regardless of scientific needs for the most efficient and effective production of useful experimental data.

Erythropoietin (EPO): A hormone produced by the kidneys that controls the production of red blood cells in the bone marrow of humans. It can be produced outside the body through **recombinant DNA technology,** and it is used therapeutically in the treatment of anemias resulting from cancer chemotherapy or chronic renal failure. It has also been used as a "blood doping" agent to increase endurance among those participating in triathlons, marathons, or long-range bicycle races by increasing the blood's oxygen-carrying capacity by increasing red blood cells.

Eschatology: Theological or philosophical study of the "end times" or "last things" on Earth, especially prominent in Christian theology. Modern Christian ethics has given much attention to the interpretation of Jesus' moral sayings and admonitions in light of his (and the early Christian churches') anticipation of the end of the known world and the incoming "Kingdom of God." Thus, for many Christians present moral obligation must be measured with reference to what Jesus has said about the conditions, promises, and requirements of that kingdom. In a broader and more general sense, eschatological expectations regarding divine intents for human futures may be considered in assessing the appropriateness of human future-planning measures such as genetic determination (via **eugenic** or **genetic engineering** efforts to "shape" future generations) or deliberate alteration of "natural" lifespans via anti-aging drugs.

Ethical relativism: See **relativism, ethical**

Ethics: In general, the study or examination of morality and moral life. The term is also used to refer to that branch of philosophy or theology dedicated to the study of morality. Several major approaches to the study of morality are encompassed under the broad term "ethics." Perhaps the best-known approach is normative ethics, which attempts to identify those moral norms, values, or traits that should be accepted as standards or guides for moral behavior and moral judgments. Practical or **applied ethics** is that aspect of normative ethics that seeks to discern the implications or directions of those accepted moral standards or guides in particular areas of moral life. Thus, bioethics, business ethics, judicial ethics, and ministerial ethics are all forms of practical or applied normative ethics, dealing with moral questions or quandaries arising in particular professional or policy areas of life. Another approach to ethics, descriptive ethics, is not normative or prescriptive in its efforts but is instead, much like the social sciences, a factual examination of the moral behavior and belief of persons or groups. It does not seek to answer moral questions about what ought to be done or judged; rather, it seeks empirical knowledge about what is believed and acted upon in the moral lives of persons as well as what causal factors may explain why those moral views are held. A third major approach to the study of morality is metaethics, which seeks to explore and describe the meaning of moral concepts, moral language, and forms of moral reasoning. For example, metaethics may explore whether social morality is emotive or rational, objective or subjective. Or it may examine the meaning of moral terms such as "value," "responsibility," "virtue," "principle," or "rights." It also includes the study of moral epistemology (i.e., theories of the sources and forms of moral knowledge) and forms or methods of moral reasoning and **justification.**

Ethics committee: See **institutional ethics committee**

Ethics of care: See **care, ethics of**

Eugenics: Social movements, programs, and policies designed to "improve" the **gene pool** through intentional human action. Beginning in the early twentieth century eugenics policies of various nations sought to decrease the number of persons born with hereditary illnesses and disabilities and to increase the number of persons born with "desirable" heritable traits. (A major center of eugenics research and data collection in the United States was the Cold Spring Harbor Laboratory in New York, where noted eugenicists Charles B. Davenport and Henry H. Laughlin maintained the "Eugenics Record Office" from 1910 until 1940 and advocated public policies that would advance eugenics goals.) Programs and policies of *negative* eugenics were designed to discourage or prevent reproduction by those deemed to be genetically unhealthy or "unfit" (i.e., those seen to be carriers of negative traits or conditions that might be inherited by any of their offspring). Programs of *positive* eugenics were established to encourage and enable the maximal level of reproduction by those deemed to be most "fit" or who bore the most socially desirable heritable traits. In the United States, many state statutes based on negative eugenics, specifically those allowing sterilization of persons diagnosed with certain mental and medical conditions deemed to be heritable, were upheld by the U.S. Supreme Court in the ***Buck v. Bell*** case (1927). Various proposals based in positive eugenics also advocated the establishment of **germplasm banks,** repositories of frozen sperm and ova from those deemed genetically most "fit," healthy, or intelligent, which would allow for fertilization of the ova of those most "fit" with the sperm of those most "fit" to produce superior offspring. Particularly in Western countries, social acceptance of eugenics policies and laws waned considerably in light of the draconian eugenics policies carried out by Adolph Hitler and the National Socialist regime in Germany. However, many argue that the selective reproductive choices now made available to potential parents through prenatal and even preimplantation genetic diagnosis have ushered in a new era of eugenical selection, albeit on a more personalized basis.

Euphenics: Interventions, procedures, and treatments intended to alter the outward symptoms or expression (**phenotype**) of genetic disorders without changing the organism's genetic constitution (**genotype**) that gives rise to those symptoms. Euphenics may involve medical or surgical treatment, dietary alteration, change in physical exercise or activity, and so on, to ameliorate otherwise deleterious manifestations of a genetic disease or disorder. So, for example, children born with the genetic disease phenylketonuria (PKU) can be treated euphenically by withholding significant levels of the amino acid phenylalanine, which their bodies cannot metabolize, from their diets.

Euthanasia: (From the Greek for "good death.") The practice of intentionally bringing about the death of an individual in a (relatively) peaceful or painless manner to prevent extended suffering or a prolonged dying process for that individual. *Active* euthanasia, sometimes referred to as "mercy killing," involves the use of drugs or other lethal means to cause the peaceful death of the individual being euthanized. *Passive* euthanasia is a form of "letting die" or "allowed death" in which death is intentionally brought about by withholding or withdrawing some form of treatment that could otherwise sustain life. Some commentators limit usage of the term "euthanasia" solely to what is described here as "active euthanasia." Because "euthanasia" is by definition intended to provide a good or benefit to the one being euthanized, the term is often qualified according to the degree of that person's voluntary request for it. *Voluntary* euthanasia occurs only with the informed request and consent of the person being euthanized. *Nonvoluntary* euthanasia occurs without the informed request or consent of that person because he has not made a request or is incompetent or too young to understand and give consent. *Involuntary* euthanasia occurs contrary to the wishes of the person being euthanized, or at least without seeking his consent or agreement. While voluntary active euthanasia is illegal throughout the United States, it has been legally accepted in several countries, most notably the Netherlands and Belgium.

Experimentation, medical: The application of any new or untested medical intervention carried out to produce measurable data regarding its effects, side effects, duration of effect, and so on. In contrast to medical therapy, which includes those diagnostic and treatment modalities whose primary purpose is to restore or maintain health, prolong life or relieve suffering, medical experimentation has the primary aim of contributing to generalizable scientific knowledge about the physiological, chemical, or psychological functioning of human beings (or animals) and the influence of particular treatment modalities upon that functioning. Experimentation involving human subjects may take the form of therapeutic research or non-therapeutic research. Therapeutic research, generally involving subjects who have some pathology or illness for which treatment is the issue under investigation, has the twin aim of generating useful medical knowledge while also (hopefully) benefiting the patient-subjects by identifying a superior form of treatment for their condition. Nontherapeutic research, usually involving healthy volunteer subjects, is concerned solely with yielding experimental data and is not aimed at providing any therapy for the subjects. The most common form of medical research protocol is the randomized clinical trial (RCT), in which subjects are randomly assigned to one of the two or more treatment "arms" of the study (i.e., groups of subjects receiving a particular medical intervention, or lack thereof) so that the effects experienced by those in each treatment arm can be carefully compared to the effects of interventions in other treatment arms of the trial.

Extrachromosomal DNA: DNA that is located within a cell but outside the chromosomes found in the cell nucleus. It is also known as extranuclear DNA. In humans, extrachromosomal DNA is generally found in the **mitochondria.** While chromosomal DNA is the major factor in determining the development of a human organism, mitochondrial DNA can also influence that development.

Extracorporeal membrane oxygenation (ECMO):   A technology, similar to heart-lung "bypass" procedures, in which the blood can be provided with oxygen (and removal of carbon dioxide) via mechanical means outside the body. (A more recent term for this procedure is ECLS, or extracorporeal life support.) In the ECMO procedure, cannulae (tubes) are placed into major blood vessels and blood is pumped through a "membrane oxygenator," which imitates the natural gas-exchange (oxygen for carbon dioxide) function of the lungs. There are two major forms of ECMO: venovenous (VV), in which blood is pumped out of and then back into a major vein, replacing lung function only; and venoarterial (VA), in which blood is pumped out of a major artery and back into a major vein, replacing not only the lungs' ventilatory function but also the heart's pumping function. ECMO's primary purpose is to provide respiratory (or cardiorespiratory) support in cases where the lungs or heart (or both) are too diseased or underdeveloped to perform their normal functions or are in need of a "rest period" for healing before resuming their normal functions. Because of its great complexity, expense, and potential medical complications, ECMO is generally considered a "last resort" intervention. Its most common usage is for premature infants in pulmonary (lung) distress.

"Extraordinary" and "ordinary" means of treatment: A distinction, first developed in Catholic moral theology beginning in the sixteenth century, regarding moral obligations to provide (or accept) various forms of life-prolonging treatment in the face of serious, life-threatening conditions. The term "extraordinary" does not mean *unusual* but rather *morally optional*, while the term "ordinary" means *morally obligatory*. In general terms, "ordinary" means of preserving life have been described as those interventions that have a reasonable prospect of benefiting the patient and that provide more benefit than the burdens they may produce for the patient. Conversely, any intervention that would have no reasonable prospect of benefiting the patient, or that would be more burdensome than beneficial for the particular patient in question, would be considered "extraordinary." Although these two historical criteria (prospect of benefit, calculus of burdens versus benefit) have become prominent base points for most contemporary discussions of the ethics of withholding or withdrawing life-prolonging treatment, interpretation of their precise meanings has been controversial. Even within the Catholic tradition, for instance, there are differences of opinion as to whether the "benefit" to be sought might be simply prolongation of physical life or whether it must include consciousness, relationality, and the capacity to seek "spiritual goods" on the part of the patient. Differences also arise, of course, as to the sorts of "burdens" (physical, emotional, economic, etc.) that might be seen to override the benefit of prolonged life. (See, e.g., Michael Panicola, "Catholic Teaching on Prolonging Life: Setting the Record Straight," *Hastings Center Report* 31, no. 6 [2001]: 14–25.)

❧ **F** ❧

Family planning: See **natural family planning**

FAS: See **fetal alcohol syndrome**

Feeding tube: A term used to describe several devices that can be used to deliver nutrition or hydration into the stomach of a person who is unable to chew, swallow, or otherwise consume food and liquids in the "normal" manner. (See **PEG tube, nasogastric tube**)

Female genital mutilation: A term used to describe the practice (in some cultures) of removing the female clitoris (known as clitoridectomy, or "female circumcision") and the labia minora, in addition to sewing together the labia majora. This practice has been condemned by many societies as being cruel or barbaric and as leading to organ damage, infections, urinary incontinence, and complications in childbirth. (See **infibulation**)

Feminist ethics: A family of ethical theories, perspectives, and approaches to moral reasoning rooted in the insights and commitments of modern forms of feminism. In general, feminism is committed to equality among all persons regardless of gender, and to mutuality in human relationships. It includes a particular concern for the well-being of women and for the inclusion of women's experiences in any understanding of what well-being and good life might be for all persons. It is opposed to beliefs, attitudes, behaviors, ideologies, and policies that establish or reinforce discrimination on the basis of gender, and it is particularly opposed to historical structures of patriarchy. Feminist ethics, then, includes a commitment to challenge male bias (based in reflection upon male experience exclusively) in inherited traditions of ethical theory and discourse. This commitment also includes the aims of morally critiquing traditions, practices, and actions that perpetuate the subordination of women; identifying moral means of resisting them; and presenting moral alternatives that promote women's full equality and personhood. Feminist ethical theories do not take one single form or employ any single methodology. They may differ in terms of their analyses of root causes of women's subordination and the best strategy for correcting it (as in differences between radical, socialist, and liberal feminist ethics, for example). They may also differ in their employment or rejection of different theories of moral justification, such as **utilitarianism, deontology, virtue ethics, casuistry,** an **ethics of care,** and so on. All feminist ethics, however, share a firm commitment to focus on women's experience as their primary source of moral insight. (See, e.g., Susan Sherwin, *No Longer Patient: Feminist Ethics and Health Care* [Philadelphia: Temple University Press, 1992], and Virginia Held, *Feminist Morality: Transforming Culture, Society, and Politics* [Chicago: University of Chicago Press, 1993].)

Fertilization: The fusion of **gametes** to form a new organism of the same species but with a new and unique genetic identity. In humans, fertilization involves the fusion of a **spermatozoon** with an **ovum,** leading to the combination of **chromosomes** from both of their nuclei, resulting in a **diploid** organism (a **zygote**) that, given favorable conditions, then begins the process of **embryonic development.**

Fetal alcohol syndrome (FAS): An array of permanent and often severe birth defects in an infant resulting from her mother's consumption of alcohol during pregnancy. These defects commonly include brain damage; facial deformities; delayed physical and emotional development; and deficits in reasoning ability, memory, and attention span. Research estimates that fetal exposure to alcohol is the most common cause of mental retardation in Western nations.

Fetal germ cells (FG): See **embryonic germ cells**

Fetal reduction (or selective reduction): A form of **abortion** in which the number of fetuses is reduced in a pregnancy involving multiple fetuses. This procedure is usually elected because of concerns about the medical complications often arising in multifetal pregnancies (e.g., premature birth, low birth weights) and most often involves "reducing" the number of fetuses down to two or even one. In many cases it is also carried out in conjunction with prior genetic testing of the multiple fetuses to selectively reduce those with the greater chance of genetic disease or defect. The procedure is generally carried out between weeks 9 and 12 of pregnancy and usually involves injecting the selected fetuses with chemicals to cause death.

Fetal tissue transplant: A procedure in which tissue from an aborted fetus is removed and transplanted into the diseased or damaged tissue of a recipient to augment or replace the function of that targeted tissue.

Fetus: In medical terminology, the developing human organism after the eighth week of **embryonic development.** (In legal terminology, "fetus" refers to the developing human organism from the completion of implantation in the uterus up until birth.)

Follicle, ovarian (or Graafian follicle):   Spherical aggregation of cells in the ovary containing an **ovum** (egg cell). At ovulation the follicle ruptures and the ovum is released.

Formalism: In ethical theory, a type of **deontology** in which an action is judged to be right if it is in accord with a moral rule and wrong if it violates a moral rule.

Formulary, pharmaceutical: A roster of drugs and other pharmaceutical preparations accepted for use in a particular institution, in a multi-institution organization, or by a regional or national government.

Fragile X syndrome: A genetic disorder caused by a **mutation** of a gene (FMR1) on the X chromosome. This gene codes for the production of a protein necessary for development of the brain; the mutation causes diminished production of that protein. Fragile X syndrome is the most common form of inherited mental impairment and is the most common known cause of autism. (See also **disorder, genetic**)

Frontal lobes: An area of the brain located at the front of each of the brain's cerebral hemispheres (the two "halves" of the upper brain). The frontal lobes have been found to be involved in language use, memory, problem solving, motor function, socialization, sexual behavior, impulse control, judgment, and spontaneity. Damage to frontal lobes can be manifest in impulsiveness, inability to plan and execute complex tasks, and other cognitive problems. Deliberate, surgical damaging of the frontal lobes, or severing their connections with the limbic system of the brain (known as prefrontal

lobotomy or **leukotomy**) was introduced in the early twentieth century as a treatment for depression, schizophrenia, and
various other mental conditions. This procedure has been
largely abandoned in recent decades.

Futility, medical: A judgment that a particular medical
intervention is unlikely to provide any significant benefit
for the patient. This judgment may be quantitative, meaning that there is little or no chance that the intervention can
achieve its intended therapeutic effect, or it may be qualita-
tive, meaning that the therapeutic effect the intervention can
achieve is not beneficial to the patient in question. There is
wide agreement that health care providers and organizations
have no moral obligation to provide treatment that is "futile"
in the sense of being "impossible to bring about" (reflecting the Kantian claim that "ought implies can"). Yet there
is much controversy regarding judgments of "futile" in the
sense of "unlikely to provide benefit" because there may be
great differences among persons regarding their own evalua-
tions of what kinds of benefit are worthy of pursuit or within
what range of statistical possibility.

ᔓ **G** ᔓ

Gamete (or germ cell): A **spermatozoon** (sperm) or **ovum** (egg) cell.

Gamete donation: The collection of **gametes** (sperm or ova) from one individual to be used for reproductive purposes by another individual (or individuals).

Gamete intrafallopian transfer (GIFT): A procedure in which sperm and ova are mixed together and then instilled artificially in a woman's fallopian tube to promote fertilization and pregnancy. (See **assisted reproductive technology**)

Gametopathy: A congenital malformation or disorder caused by chromosomal abnormalities in the sperm or ovum from which an individual was conceived.

Gene: The basic functional and physical unit of heredity consisting of an organized sequence of **DNA** nucleotides at a particular position on a particular **chromosome.** This DNA sequence provides the blueprint for the production of proteins that will form the structures of all parts of the cell (and organism).

Gene expression: The process in which a gene's coding sequence is converted into the structures that exist and operate within the cell (and organism in general). Also, the phenotypic manifestation of a characteristic (such as hair color or eye color) encoded by a particular gene.

Gene pool: The sum total of all the genes and variations of those genes (**alleles**) found in a particular population or collection of organisms of the same species. The human gene pool, then, consists of all the allelic variations of genes present in the population of human beings.

Generic drugs: Drugs that are produced as the pharmacological equivalents (in chemical structure, dosage, absorption and excretion, etc.) of existing brand–name drugs. Because they are essentially copies of existing pharmaceutical products, they are generally produced only after the patent for the original drug has expired or otherwise been deemed invalid. Generic drugs are usually priced lower than their brand–name counterparts because their manufacturers did not have to bear the original costs of research and development for the brand–name drugs.

Gene therapy: The insertion of DNA sequences (genes) into cells or tissues to treat a disease, especially a hereditary disease. The purpose of gene therapy is to replace a mutant or disease-producing gene **allele** with a more functional allele at the same chromosomal location. Generally, the "normal" allele is delivered into the cell by means of a **vector** or carrier molecule, usually a virus that has been altered to carry normal human DNA. Gene therapy undertaken thus far has been somatic cell gene therapy because its "target" cells have been body cells other than sperm and ova. Theoretically, however, germline gene therapy would also be possible, introducing new gene alleles into the genetic makeup of sperm and ova cells. Germline gene therapy is somewhat more controversial in that it would alter the genetic complement (**genome**) not only of the individual undergoing therapy but also of any offspring he might produce.

Genetically modified organism (GMO):   An organism whose genetic material has been altered via genetic technology, particularly **recombinant DNA technology.** Many plants, for instance, have been genetically modified to make them more resistant to disease or insect attack or to maximize their relative nutrient value (to animals or human consumers).

Genetic code: The messenger **RNA** nucleotide sequence, coded in triplets (codons) and sequenced according to its pairing with the **DNA** sequence in a **gene,** that determines the sequence of amino acids in the synthesis of proteins (and thus the formation of cell structures, tissues, organs, etc.).

Genetic determinism: The idea that certain physical and behavioral traits are expressions of, and thus are necessarily determined by, the presence of particular genes or groups of genes in that individual's cells. Certain genetic diseases (e.g., **sickle cell anemia, Tay-Sachs disease, Down syndrome**) provide clear examples of this. There is much controversy surrounding claims of the genetic determination of certain traits such as risk–attraction, predispositions toward violent behavior, and sexual orientation. (See **determinism**)

Genetic discrimination: Prejudice, disfavor, or restrictions placed against persons who have or are likely to develop an inherited disease or disorder.

Genetic disorder: A condition caused by the abnormal expression of one or more genes in an individual, leading to abnormal physical or mental structure or function. Genetic disorders may be caused by abnormal numbers of chromosomes (see **aneuploidy**), by spontaneous mutations of genes that effect their expression, or by inheritance of defective or disordered genes from one's parents. Some hereditary genetic disorders are caused by a defective **recessive gene,** in which case the gene must be inherited in the chromosomes from both parents to produce the abnormal traits in the offspring. Examples would include cystic fibrosis, Tay-Sachs disease, and sickle cell anemia. Conversely, a defective dominant gene will produce the abnormal traits in the offspring if the gene is inherited in the chromosomes of only one parent. Huntington's disease would be an example of an autosomal (i.e., caused by genes on a non–sex chromosome) dominant genetic disorder. Some other genetic disorders—e.g., hemophilia, color blindness, and forms of male infertility—are caused by defects on the X or Y sex chromosomes and thus are known as sex-linked disorders. While some disorders are single-gene disorders (i.e., disorders due to a "mistake" at single gene location on a given chromosome), others are multifactoral or polygenic, meaning that they result from the effects of multiple genes and from gene expression in combination with environmental and lifestyle factors. Diabetes mellitus and some forms of heart disease would be examples of multifactoral genetic disorders. While the effects of some genetic disorders are present from birth, late-onset disorders may not become manifest until late childhood, adulthood, or even old age (even though genetic testing for these disorders may be possible from conception onward). Examples of **late-onset disorders** include **Huntington's disease,** Alzheimer's disease, and some forms of heart disease.

Genetic engineering: Altering the genetic material within a cell or organism to allow it to perform new functions or produce new substances.

Genetic fingerprinting: See **DNA fingerprinting**

Genetic intervention: A general term for intentional manipulation or alteration of an organism's genetic material, as in **gene therapy,** to bring about some desired alteration in that organism's structure or function.

Genetic linkage: See **linkage, genetic**

Genetics: The science or study of **genes, heredity,** and variation among organisms.

Genetic screening: Testing a group or population of persons to identify those having or carrying a genetic trait for (and thus able to pass on to offspring) a hereditary disease or abnormality.

Genetic testing: The analysis of an individual's **DNA** and **RNA,** and the chromosome structures, proteins, and other metabolites in cells to diagnose various genetic or chromosomal disorders or diseases (or carrier status), to determine the individual's sex, or to trace her genetic ancestry.

Genetic therapy: See **gene therapy**

Gene transfer: The introduction and incorporation of new **DNA** sequences into an organism's cells, usually by means of a viral **vector.** This procedure is employed in **gene therapy.**

Genome: The total complement of genetic material in an organism. (Or, in its broader definition, "genome" can refer to the total complement of genetic material in a population of organisms of the same species—i.e., its **gene pool.**)

Genomics: The study of genes and their functions, including their interaction with one another and with other cellular, pharmacological, and environmental influences.

Genotype: The specific genetic makeup (**genome**) of an organism. One's genotype, together with environmental factors influencing genetic expression, provides the coded blueprint for one's physical appearance and function, or **phenotype.**

Germ cell: A **spermatozoon** (sperm) or **ovum** (egg) cell, also called a **gamete.**

Germinal choice: A term arising from the **eugenics** movement of the early twentieth century and referring to a program of intentional decisions to produce the most genetically superior children by bringing together sperm and ova from the most "fit" or genetically "healthy" individuals. Its most famous (or infamous) institutional manifestation came with the opening of millionaire Robert K. Graham's Repository for Germinal Choice in California in 1979. Based on a scheme first proposed by geneticist Hermann J. Muller in the 1930s, the "repository" was intended to be a sperm bank for the sperm of Nobel Prize winners. Eugenically minded women could thus choose to be impregnated with the sperm of intellectually "superior" males to produce creative, intelligent offspring.

Germline genetic therapy: The introduction of new gene alleles into the genetic makeup of sperm and ova cells. Germline gene therapy is somewhat controversial in that it alters the genetic complement (genome) not only of the individual undergoing therapy but also of any offspring he might produce. See **gene therapy.**

Germplasm bank: Early terminology connoting repositories for frozen donated sperm and ova (i.e., "sperm banks" and "ova banks") that might be thawed and used for reproductive purposes by persons who face infertility problems or who wish to avoid transmitting hereditary diseases or otherwise promote the aims of **eugenics.** An early promoter of this idea was American geneticist Hermann J. Muller in the 1930s.

Gestation: Pregnancy; the period of development of the embryo/fetus from **fertilization** and implantation until birth.

GH: See **growth hormone**

GIFT: See **gamete intrafallopian transfer**

GMO: See **genetically modified organism**

Gonads: Organs in the body that produce **gametes** (sperm and ova). The male gonads are testes; female gonads are ovaries.

Griswold v. Connecticut: Legal case argued before the U.S. Supreme Court (381 U.S. 479 [1965]) challenging a Connecticut law forbidding the distribution or use of contraceptive devices. The court's majority opinion, written by Justice William O. Douglas, struck down the Connecticut law (and similar laws in other states), claiming that it violated the "marital right to privacy" in reproductive decisions. Although this right of privacy is not found in the Bill of Rights, the opinion observed, it may be found in the "penumbras" and "emanations" of other personal rights protected by the Constitution. This claim of a right to privacy in reproductive matters became an important factor in the U.S. Supreme Court's decision in the ***Roe v. Wade*** case in 1973.

Growth hormone (GH):   Also called somatropin or somatotropin, GH is a polypeptide hormone produced in the anterior pituitary gland. Its effect is to stimulate cell reproduction and growth (height growth, bone strengthening, muscle mass increase, immune system stimulation, etc.) in humans and other vertebrate animals. Deficiency of growth hormone in the human body leads to growth retardation and short stature in children, and to diminished strength, energy, and bone mass in adults. A biosynthetic form of human growth hormone (hGH) has been produced via **recombinant DNA technology** and is widely used in therapeutic contexts. While treatment of GH deficiency via administration of recombinant hGH is widely accepted, some potential uses of hGH therapy are controversial. These include its use as an attempt to reverse the effects of aging in older adults, to enhance weight loss in persons with obesity, and to improve athletic performance and bodybuilding. Some parents, desiring athletic glory for their children, have requested its administration to those children in the hope of producing greater-than-normal height and muscle mass.

❧ **H** ❧

Haploid.   The term used to describe the number of chromosomes found in the **germ cells** (sperm or egg cells) of an individual. In human beings, the normal haploid number of chromosomes is twenty-three, whereas the **diploid** number, found in all other body cells, is forty-six.

Harvard criteria for irreversible coma: A set of clinical characteristics of "irreversible coma" proposed as evidence of whole brain death: unreceptivity and unresponsivity, no movements or (unassisted) breathing, and no reflexes. A flat electroencephalogram (EEG) should provide corroboration of this diagnosis, and potentially reversible neurological conditions, such as those caused by hypothermia or barbiturate overdosage, must be ruled out. (See **brain death**)

Health maintenance organization (HMO):   A form of **managed care organization (MCO)** in the United States that provides health insurance coverage by meeting the health care needs of its members through hospitals, clinicians, and other providers under contract with the HMO. Treatment provided in an HMO usually follows a set of care guidelines applied throughout the organization by its contracted care providers. The original concept of an HMO focused upon "maintenance" of the health of its members, stressing routine screening tests and other preventive measures and thus ostensibly avoiding the need for expensive treatment interventions later on. Most HMOs require members to select a primary care physician (PCP) from its roster of contracted providers, who then serves as a "gatekeeper" and who must provide referral for all other health services the member may need. HMOs also employ "utilization review" and "case management" to identify forms of treatment that may be unnecessary, ineffective, or beyond the contracted specifications for care provision.

Hedonism, hedonic calculus: A form of reasoning in which the production of pleasure is the central focus and goal. As an ethical theory, hedonism might be expressed in the claim, "whatever causes the greatest pleasure is right." This view assumes that all actions can be measured and assessed on the basis of how much pleasure or pain they produce. The hedonist chooses a course of action by weighing (in a "hedonic calculus") the relative degrees of pleasure and pain that can be predicted to result from each available alternative action, then choosing that one action that will produce the greatest pleasure and the least pain. Hedonism may be egoistic, focused upon maximizing pleasure for oneself alone, or it may be altruistic, focused upon maximizing pleasure for all persons affected by one's choices. The two earliest proponents of **utilitarianism,** Jeremy Bentham and John Stuart Mill, are often referred to as hedonistic utilitarians because their understanding of "utility" (producing the greatest good for the greatest number) was usually expressed in terms of the maximization of pleasure or happiness.

Hemizygote: A **diploid** organism (having paired **chromosomes,** one set inherited from each parent) in which one chromosome segment or one **allele** at a particular gene location is missing. For example, the human male is a hemizygote for all genes contained on the X chromosome because males normally inherit only one X chromosome and thus are not diploid for that particular chromosome.

Hemoglobin: The iron-containing metalloprotein in the red cells (erythrocytes) of blood that transports oxygen. Oxygen binds to hemoglobin in the lungs and is transported to muscle and other bodily tissues.

Herbalism (phytotherapy):   An "alternative" or "complementary" form of medical practice based in the use of plants and plant derivatives. Evidence exists of medicinal use of plants from more than 60,000 years ago. Some contemporary "standard" pharmaceutical products (e.g., quinine, digitalis, opioid narcotics) have been used as herbal remedies for many centuries.

Heredity: In biological teims, the genetic transfer of biological characteristics from parent to offspring.

Heritability: The proportion of the variation among **phenotypes** in a population that can be attributed to the variation in **genotypes** in that population. Several factors can influence variation among phenotypes (the observable characteristics of individuals), and heritability studies examine the relative degree to which genetic differences account for phenotypic variations within a population.

Hermaphrodite: An organism that possesses both male and female sex organs during its life.

Heroic treatment: An expression used to convey the judgment that a particular form of (life-prolonging) treatment goes beyond the normal obligations of care or is considered morally **extraordinary.** See **"extraordinary" and "ordinary" means of treatment.**

Heterograft (or xenograft):   Organs, tissues, or cells transplanted from an organism of one species to an organism of another species (e.g., from a pig to a human being). (See **transplantation, organ and tissue**)

Heteronomy: The condition of being under the control or domination, especially with respect to the power of decision or choice, of some authority (human or divine) outside the self. Heteronomy is generally taken to mean the opposite of genuine **autonomy.** (See **autonomy**)

Heterozygote: An organism that contains more than one **allele** at the same position on paired or multiple homologous (related) **chromosomes.** Humans, for example, are **diploid** (having paired sets of chromosomes in each **somatic** cell, one set inherited from each parent). Thus, a human heterozygote for a particular gene will have two different versions (alleles) of that gene on the two different paired chromosomes containing that gene location.

Heterozygous: Having more than one version (**allele**) of a gene at the same location on paired or multiple chromosomes (in organisms whose cells contain more than one set of chromosomes). (See **heterozygote**)

Hippocrates: An ancient Greek physician (circa 460–370 BCE) on the Island of Cos, generally regarded as the father of [Western] medicine. The Hippocratic school of medicine that he founded revolutionized medical practice in ancient Greece and helped establish medicine as a distinct professional field. Hippocrates and his physician-followers left a collection of writings collectively known as the Hippocratic Corpus, which includes the famous Hippocratic oath still in use in many medical school graduation ceremonies. (See, e.g., Ludwig Edelstein, *Ancient Medicine* [Baltimore: Johns Hopkins University Press, 1967].)

Histocompatibility antigens: Proteins on the surface of cells in the body that may be recognized as either "normal" or "foreign" by the immune system. Antigens recognized as foreign (such as those in organs or tissues transplanted from another individual) trigger production of **antibodies** by the immune system to attack the foreign proteins. Human histocompatibility antigens are called HLA (**human leukocyte antigens**). (See **transplantation, organ and tissue**)

HIV: See **human immunodeficiency virus**

HLA: See **human leukocyte antigens**

HMO: See **health maintenance organization; managed care**

Holistic medicine: An approach to health care and maintenance that emphasizes extension beyond traditional **allopathic** medicine to include "alternative" or "complementary" medicine and "natural healing" techniques. According to one definition by the Canadian Holistic Medical Association, holistic medicine is "a system of health care which fosters a cooperative relationship among all those involved, leading towards optimal attainment of the physical, mental, emotional, social and spiritual aspects of health. . . . It emphasizes the need to look at the whole person, including analysis of physical, nutritional, environmental, emotional, social, spiritual and lifestyle values. It encompasses all stated modalities of diagnosis and treatment including drugs or surgery if no safe alternative exists. Holistic medicine focuses on education and responsibility for personal efforts to achieve balance and well being."

Hominization: See **animation**

Homograft (or allograft):   Tissue or organ taken from a donor organism and transplanted into a recipient organism of the same species but of different genetic makeup, thus requiring suppression of the recipient's immune system to prevent rejection of the graft. (See **transplantation**)

Homologous recombination: The "swapping" of fragments of **DNA** between two paired chromosomes. Also called "DNA crossover."

Homozygote: An organism that contains the same version or **allele** of a gene at the same position on paired or multiple homologous (related) **chromosomes.** Humans are **diploid,** having paired sets of chromosomes in each **somatic** cell, one set inherited from each parent. So a human homozygote for a particular gene will have the very same version (allele) of that gene on the two different paired chromosomes containing that gene location.

Homozygous: Having the same version (**allele**) of a particular gene at the same location on paired or multiple chromosomes (in organisms whose cells contain more than one set of chromosomes). (See **homozygote**)

Hospice: In older terminology, a place of shelter or rest, usually maintained by a religious order for pilgrims or other travelers. In contemporary usage, the term refers to a program, organization, or institution that provides **palliative care**

and other support services (spiritual, psychological, social) rather than curative or life-prolonging interventions to persons who are terminally ill. Hospice care may be provided in institutional settings or, more commonly, in a patient's home. The modern hospice movement began in the United Kingdom with the establishment of St. Christopher's Hospice by Dr. Cicely Saunders in 1967.

Hospital ethics committee: See **institutional ethics committee**

Humanae vitae: (Latin meaning "human life") Title of a papal encyclical issued by Pope Paul VI in 1968. Subtitled "On the Regulation of Birth," *Humanae vitae* reaffirmed traditional Roman Catholic teaching regarding abortion, birth control, family planning, and other related issues. It is perhaps best known for its firm reassertion of the **natural law** argument against any use of artificial contraception: that procreation is the natural end or purpose of sexual activity, therefore each act of sexual intercourse must at least be open to the possibility of conception. (In this reasoning, **natural family planning** methods could be acceptable under certain circumstances.)

Human Genome Organization (HUGO):   An international organization established in 1989 and involved in the **Human Genome Project.** The Gene Nomenclature Committee of HUGO is working to assign unique gene names and symbols to all human genes.

Human Genome Project (HGP):   Initially named the Human Genome Initiative, the project began as several programs initiated in the 1980s by the U.S. Department of Energy to identify all the 20,000–25,000 **genes** comprising human **DNA;** determine the sequences of the 3 billion base pairs that make up human DNA; create databases to store this information;

improve means of data analysis; make related technologies available to the private sector; and address ethical, legal, and social issues (**ELSI**) that may arise as newly available genetic information is disseminated. Ultimately a joint national effort coordinated by the Department of Energy and the National Institutes of Health (and funded at more than $3 billion by the U.S. government) the Human Genome Project was completed in thirteen years (in 2003) and also involved contributions from the United Kingdom, Germany, France, Japan, China, and other nations.

Human immunodeficiency virus (HIV):   (Formerly known as HTLV-III and lymphadenopathy-associated virus) A **retrovirus** that is the cause of AIDS (acquired human immunodeficiency syndrome), a syndrome in which the body's immune system fails, leading to serious opportunistic infections. The HIV virus attacks important parts of the immune system (CD4+ T cells, macrophages, dendritic cells) and organs such as the heart, kidneys, and brain. It can be transmitted when a bodily fluid (blood, semen, breast milk, vaginal secretions) containing the virus comes into contact with a mucous membrane. The virus was first identified in 1983.

Humanism: A broad collection of moral philosophies that emphasize the dignity and value of human beings and the capacity to discern right and wrong through appeal to universal human qualities and characteristics, especially rationality. Modern humanisms appear in both secular and religious forms. Secular humanism—a term frequently used disparagingly by some conservative religious groups—emphasizes the primacy of human value (and valuing) and rejects appeals to theistic religious belief or the existence of divine powers. Religious humanisms, especially Christian and Jewish humanisms, emphasize the connection and complementarity between revealed religious knowledge and experientially affirmed knowledge of the good, the right, and the authentically human.

Human leukocyte antigens (HLA):   Human histocompatibility antigens. A person's HLA antigens are built from amino acids that are coded for by **genes** on chromosome 6. Because there are various **alleles** for each of those genes, a variety of forms of HLA antigens are coded for and produced within the human species. To prevent rejection of graft organs or tissues in **transplantation,** it is important to try to "match" the particular HLA types of the recipient with those of the potential donor. (Different organs and tissues have different requirements for the actual degree of closeness of the HLA match.) HLA matching is not a problem, of course, if graft donor and recipient are identical twins because they would share the same genetic endowment and thus the same HLA types. HLA matches that are much less "close" require the use of antirejection drugs to suppress the production of antibodies by the recipient's immune system. See **transplantation, organ and tissue.** (See **histocompatibility antigens**)

Human Subjects Review Board: See **institutional review board**

Huntington's disease (HD):   (Formerly known as Huntington's chorea) A rare genetic disorder characterized by a progressive development of uncontrollable body movements and breakdown of mental functions. Symptoms of the disease usually begin to appear between ages forty and fifty. It takes its name from Dr. George Huntington, who first described its symptomology in 1872. The causative gene for HD is located on human chromosome 4. The disease has an autosomal dominant form of inheritance, meaning that each offspring of an individual bearing the defective HD gene allele has a 50 percent chance of inheriting the disease. (See **autosomal disorder**)

Hydranencephaly: A **neural tube defect** in which the cerebral hemispheres are absent, and replaced by sacs of cerebrospinal fluid. (See **neural tube defect**)

Hydrocephaly: See **neural tube defect**

Hyperalimentation: A procedure for delivering the body's nutritional requirements in liquid form, usually into a major vein via a central catheter (such as a **PICC**), for persons who are unable to swallow, digest, or absorb nutrients delivered orally. Hyperalimentation solutions generally are composed of proteins, sugars, vitamins and minerals, electrolytes, and fat emulsions. Another term for hyperalimentation is TPN or total parenteral nutrition.

Hypoxia: In the body, a reduction (below what is physiologically normal) in the level of oxygen in tissues. This is usually caused by either an interruption or diminishment of oxygen-carrying blood flow to the affected tissues (also called ischemia) or by a decreased level of oxygen-transporting **hemoglobin** in the blood (as in conditions of anemia).

Hysterectomy: Surgical removal of the female uterus.

Hysterotomy abortion: **Abortion** procedure in which the fetus is removed by making an incision in the pregnant woman's abdomen and into the uterus; this is essentially an early Caesarian section delivery, albeit not resulting in live birth. (See **abortion**)

Iatrogenic: From Greek roots meaning "healer induced," a disease or adverse effect resulting from a treatment intervention by a health practitioner.

Immunodeficiency (or immune deficiency): The medical condition in which the immune system's ability to fight infections is diminished or absent. Some forms of immunodeficiency are congenital (from birth), due to heritable genetic diseases. Others are acquired, resulting from blood disorders such as multiple myeloma or chronic lymphocytic leukemia, from infectious agents such as the **HIV** virus, or from the introduction of immune-suppressing drugs to treat **autoimmune disease** or malignancies or to prevent rejection of foreign organs or tissues in **transplantation.**

Immunogen: See **antigen**

Immunoglobulins (Ig): A related group of (animal) glycoproteins that function as **antibodies** to attack invasive **antigens** in the body. All immunoglobulin molecules are composed of protein chains ("light" chains or "heavy" chains) linked together with chemical bonds. The five major (heavy chain) classes of immunoglobulins in the human body are IgG, IgA, IgD, IgE, and IgM. Igs are found in blood and tissue fluids and in various bodily secretions.

Immunosuppression: The process of deactivating or limiting the function of the body's immune system. Medically induced immunosuppression involves the use of drugs that help prevent the immune system's rejection of foreign tissues (as in organ or tissue **transplantation**) or that limit the effects of **autoimmune diseases** (such as Crohn's disease or rheumatoid arthritis). In the past, radiation was also used to suppress the body's immune responses. The first effective chemical agent identified with immunosuppressive properties was cortisone, followed in later years by azathioprine, **cyclosporine,** and other newer antirejection drugs used in transplantation contexts.

Implantation: The point at which a developing embryo becomes attached to the endometrial lining of a woman's uterus, generally seven to fourteen days after **fertilization** (see **embryonic development**). In medical terminology, "pregnancy" refers to the period following implantation (and before birth). In some cases implantation can occur in the lining of the fallopian tube, leading to **ectopic pregnancy.**

Infanticide: The practice of intentionally causing the death of an infant (by a member of the infant's own species). Human infanticide practices were common in many ancient cultures for which we have written records, including Greek, Roman, Japanese, Chinese and Indian. Reasons for infanticide have included infant deformity or illness, sex selection, population control, child sacrifice, or political domination. Ancient infanticide was often accomplished by means of deliberate malnourishment or abandonment so the child would die of exposure or starvation and dehydration. In general, modern societies hold infanticide to be both immoral and criminal.

Infibulation: In some ancient cultures, the practice of sewing together the female vaginal labia majora or male foreskin to ensure chastity. In its modern usage, the term usually refers to a practice, mostly confined to sub–Saharan African cultures and performed on pubescent females, that also includes removal of the clitoris (clitoridectomy, or "female circumcision") and the labia minora, in addition to sewing together the labia majora. This practice is often termed female genital mutilation, and has been condemned by many societies as being cruel or barbaric and as leading to organ damage, infections, urinary incontinence, and complications in childbirth.

Informed consent: In health care contexts, a legal (and moral) condition or requirement in which an individual (or, in some cases, her legitimate proxy decision maker) can be said to have given consent to receive treatment or to become a subject of research based upon clear knowledge and appreciation of the treatment or research in question and its potential implications. Generally, the concept of informed consent can be seen to have several criteria or facets: competence of the individual to understand information given and reach a reasoned decision; voluntariness in consenting, without coercion, manipulation, and so on; disclosure of information sufficient to make a reasonably informed decision (and in clinical therapy contexts, recommendation of a plan of treatment favored by the clinician and his reasons for that recommendation); comprehension by the consenter of information and recommendations disclosed; and, finally, the consenter's decision to authorize the proposed treatment plan or research participation. Legal standards for evaluating the type and quantity of information that must be disclosed in the informed consent process vary among U.S. jurisdictions between the "professional practice" (or "reasonable doctor") standard and the

"reasonable person" standard. The former assesses adequate disclosure of information based upon customary disclosure practices within the professional community while the latter focuses on what a "reasonable" patient or subject would want and need to know under the circumstances. (See, e.g., Tom L. Beauchamp and James F. Childress, *Principles of Biomedical Ethics*, 6th ed. [New York: Oxford University Press, 2009], chapter 4.) While much attention has been given to the requirement of informed consent in medical research since the Nuremburg "Doctors' Trials" in Germany in the late 1940s (and in clinical medicine since the advent of the so-called patients' rights movement of the late 1960s), there is still much debate over issues such as the validity of proxy or surrogate consents (and in what contexts), the acceptability of "implied" or "tacit" consents versus explicit consents, and the need for renewal of consents when the originally disclosed information changes.

Insemination: See **artificial insemination**

Institutional ethics committee (IEC):   A multidisciplinary committee established to consider ethical issues, concerns, and dilemmas within a health care organization or institution (hospital, clinic, nursing facility, home for the aged, etc.). IECs were proposed initially as a venue for review of decisions about withholding or limiting life-prolonging treatment in patients with terminal conditions or severe neurological damage. Eventually, however, the concept of the IEC evolved so as to include three primary purposes: (1) to educate health professionals (and, often, those they serve) about issues of concern and importance in biomedical ethics; (2) to provide a forum for reflective review and evaluation of policies within the institution that have ethical ramifications; and (3) to provide case consultation (prospective, retrospective, or both) to clarify moral issues at stake and recommend forms of resolution (and quite often providing support and encouragement for families, clinicians, and others facing difficult moral decisions). Also, while the traditional focus of IECs has been clinical ethics, more recently they have also taken on a role in **organizational ethics** relating to the business and human resource aspects of health care institutions. Generally, IECs do not supplant clinical or administrative judgment by making binding decisions regarding policy or treatment choices. Rather, their role is advisory, focusing on the procedure of providing considered, reflective, moral discourse about a policy or case rather than the outcome of making specific clinical or organizational decisions. In the United States, institutional ethics committees are one possible mechanism through which health care institutions may meet **JCAHO** procedural requirements for dealing with ethical conflicts and dilemmas relating to patients' rights and organizational ethics.

Institutional review board (IRB):   Also called a human sub jects review board, an IRB is a committee containing members of mixed backgrounds and including both scientist and nonscientist members whose task is to review and monitor biomedical and behavioral research involving human subjects. Generally, IRBs are expected to review each research **protocol** in a given institution, organization, or area before the research is begun, and then again at least once after the experiment is under way. The chief objectives of IRB reviews are to assess the scientific and ethical merit and usefulness of the research and its methods, to safeguard the well-being of research subjects, and to guarantee fully informed and voluntary participation by those subjects. In the United States, the Research Act of 1974 established the regulatory role of IRBs and mandated IRB review of all research receiving direct or indirect funding from the Department of Health and Human

Services (DHHS), which also provides regulation of IRB activities through its Office for Human Research Protections. While most IRBs operate within particular academic or clinical medical institutions, some have been established as for-profit organizations, providing contracted reviews of research protocols for commercial enterprises.

Interferons (IFNs):   A class of proteins (cytokines, a form of glycoproteins) produced by cells in the body's immune system in response to invasion by foreign bacteria, viruses, or tumor cells. There are three major classes of interferons: alpha, beta, and gamma. Interferons help regulate the body's immune and inflammatory responses, are part of its antiviral and antitumor responses, and trigger production of antibacterial cells (macrophages, natural killer lymphocytes). They have been useful therapies in the treatment of viral infections (e.g., hepatitis C) and cancer (e.g., chronic myelogenous leukemia).

Intergenerational equity: A term expressing the idea of fairness in the distribution of access to material, social, and economic benefits (as well as the assignment of related burdens) between current and future generations of persons. The concept of intergenerational equity is appealed to most frequently in discussions regarding current practices that consume or destroy nonrenewable natural resources or that create some form of indebtedness that cannot or will not be repaid by the borrowing generation but instead is left to succeeding generations. Thus, concerns about intergenerational equity are often raised in debates regarding current tax reductions that will yield large governmental deficits for the future, vast consumption of health care resources that are not being paid for by the consumer generation, and rapid depletion of fossil fuel reserves to meet current needs.

Intracytoplasmic sperm injection (ICSI):   An assisted reproductive technique in which a single sperm cell is injected into a retrieved ovum, after which the fertilized ovum (zygote) is placed in the woman's uterus or fallopian tube. (See **assisted reproductive technology**)

Intrauterine device (IUD):   A small plastic T-shaped device which can be inserted into a woman's uterus to provide contraception. Some forms of IUD contain copper while other forms are coated with slow-release hormones. IUDs do not prevent ovulation (release of an ovum or egg cell by the ovaries) but work by preventing fertilization of the ovum by sperm. Hormone-bearing IUDs also act to thicken the cervical mucosa, forming a barrier to sperm entry. IUDs also alter the endometrial lining of the uterus, preventing **implantation** of any ovum that may have been fertilized.

Intrauterine growth retardation (IUGR):   A condition in pregnancy in which a fetus's growth is significantly decreased (in medical terms, below the 10th percentile of predicted fetal weight for a fetus of that gestational age). Its most common cause is inadequate maternal–fetal blood circulation, but it may also be caused by certain infections in the uterus (e.g, cytomegalovirus or rubella) or by certain congenital defects such as Trisomy 13 or Trisomy 18. (See **aneuploidy**)

Investigational drug: A newly developed drug that is undergoing research and study but is not yet approved by government agencies to be legally marketed and sold. Investigational drugs generally are available only to those patient-subjects who are enrolled in a **clinical trial** involving that drug. However, special exceptions are made in some cases so persons who are otherwise ineligible to participate in a clinical trial may have access to "compassionate use" of an investigational drug that shows great promise of prolonging survival or improving quality of life.

In vitro fertilization (IVF):   A form of **assisted reproductive technology (ART)** in which sperm and ova (egg) cells are mixed together in a laboratory dish to allow for **fertilization,** after which the resulting **zygote** is transferred to a woman's uterus with the intent of resulting in pregnancy. "In vitro" is Latin for "in glass," although the procedure usually does not involve any glass instruments. (See **assisted reproductive technology**)

In vivo: Latin for "in the living," refers to observation or experiment involving a complete, living organism (as opposed to "in vitro" or laboratory observation or experiment involving organs, tissues, cells, proteins, etc., taken from an organism). Clinical **experimentation** involving human or animal subjects would be examples of in vivo research.

IRB: See **institutional review board**

Ischemia: Insufficient supply of blood to a bodily organ, tissue, or part, usually due to restriction or blockage of blood vessels.

IUD: See **intrauterine device**

IUGR: See **intrauterine growth retardation**

IVF: See **in vitro fertilization**

∽ J ∽

JCAHO: Joint Commission on Accreditation of Health-care Organizations—a private, nonprofit organization that identifies standards for health care organizations and applies those standards in evaluating and accrediting those organizations (including hospitals, ambulatory care clinics, behavioral health institutions, home care and long-term care organizations, and laboratories). JCAHO accreditation requirements for hospitals include standards relating to **organizational ethics,** patients' **rights,** and patient responsibilities. Hospitals are required, for example, to have procedures and mechanisms in place for dealing with ethical dilemmas and conflicts of interest in patient care, treatment, and services and in the organization's business practices. A functioning **institutional ethics committee (IEC)** provides one such mechanism for organized ethical reflection, as does an ethics consultation service. (For specific standards, see *Hospital Accreditation Standards* [Oakbrook Terrace, IL: Joint Commission Resources, 2008].)

Justice: In modern ethical discourse, the moral principle that relates to proper "balance" or allotment among persons or groups. Much contemporary discussion of the meaning of justice is rooted in Aristotle's attempts to define it, especially in Book V of his *Nicomachean Ethics* (trans. Martin Ostwald, New York: Bobbs-Merrill, 1962). For Aristotle, justice is understood primarily as a state of character, or virtue—a developed set of good habits, attitudes, and dispositions. He goes on to distinguish between "general" or "complete" justice, on the one hand, and "partial" or "particular" justice on the other. General justice is "complete virtue or excellence . . . in relation to our fellow men"—generally synonymous with "righteousness" or "honesty," perhaps. Partial justice is subdivided by Aristotle into the justice of distribution (of honors, wealth, or other social goods or benefits) and the justice of rectification in transactions (involving "making right" violations of "voluntary transactions" or contracts, and rectifying "involuntary transactions" such as theft or murder through punishments, etc.). Aristotle's description of partial justice, in particular, has given rise to four major modern applications of justice: distributive justice, retributive justice, compensatory justice, and rectificatory justice. Distributive justice involves, as Aristotle suggested, the proper or fair **allocation** of material and social benefits and burdens among persons and among groups in society. (His guiding, formal principle is that we should give to each person what they deserve or "treat equals equally and unequals unequally," but he never specified particular criteria as appropriate bases for recognizing or assessing relevant equalities among persons.) Retributive justice concerns balancing injuries or crimes with appropriate punishments (and, possibly, noble or heroic acts with appropriate rewards). Compensatory justice deals with balancing particular burdens borne by persons in the past with particular benefits in the present or future. And rectificatory justice relates to the rebalancing of interests among parties when transactions or contracts have been violated or fraudulently conceived or executed. In the discourse of health care ethics, distributive justice and compensatory justice are frequently addressed in a variety of contexts. Compensatory justice has been, for example, the source of impetus for the development of the Veterans Administration health care system in the United States and was the original basis for the development of affirmative action programs, especially with respect to preferential hiring policies. Issues of distributive justice infuse all aspects of the health care system. Perhaps the most fundamental question of distributive justice in health care—and the most nagging, in recent U.S. history—is, "Do all persons have positive **rights** to health care access, and, if so, to what extent?" But all societies must address questions of distributive justice at the levels of both **macroallocation** decisions (e.g., how much funding should be allocated to Medicare and Medicaid programs, how much for public health efforts, environmental clean-up programs) and **microallocation** decisions (e.g., which patients in organ failure will be placed on transplant waiting lists, and which will receive scarce transplantable organs when they become available). (See, e.g., Tom Beauchamp and James F. Childress, *Principles of Biomedical Ethics,* 6th ed. [New York: Oxford University Press, 2009], chapter 7).

Justification, moral: The process of providing more good reasons (both acceptable and relevant) for one moral conclusion or course of action as opposed to any clear alternative conclusion or course of action.

೫ K ೫

Karyotype: The complete set of all **chromosomes** in the cell nucleus of an organism. In the human organism, the normal **diploid** number of chromosomes (in a **somatic** cell) is forty-six chromosomes (two times twenty-three) plus two sex chromosomes (XX in a female, XY in a male). Karyotyping, the process of displaying the set of chromosomes, generally shows the chromosomes lined up in matched pairs and ordered by size. The karyotypes can then be examined for visible aberrations on particular chromosomes, chromosomes that are missing or appear in greater than normal numbers (see **aneuploidy**), and certain other aspects of the organism's **genotype** such as its sex.

⌇ L ⌇

Laparoscopy: A surgical procedure in which cameras and other instruments are introduced into the abdominal cavity through small holes created in the abdominal wall. Laparoscopy involves a much smaller incision into the abdominal wall (and less scarring) than the more traditional **laparotomy** procedure.

Laparotomy: A surgical procedure that involves an incision (surgical cutting) through the abdominal wall to gain access to the organs within the abdominal cavity for repair or removal of abdominal organs or tissues.

Late-onset disorder: Diseases or disorders whose symptoms do not appear from birth but become manifest only later in life. For example, Alzheimer's disease and **Huntington's disease** are both late-onset disorders. (See **disorder, genetic**)

LD50:   Abbreviation for "lethal dose, 50 percent," a term used in toxicology to indicate the dosage of a toxic substance or radiation required to kill 50 percent of the organisms in a given test population (usually laboratory animals) exposed to it. LD50 figures are often used as measures of the relative or comparative toxicity of various substances and are frequently expressed (at least for chemical toxins) in terms of mass of the chemical substance relative to body mass of the organism affected by it (e.g., grams or milligrams of a drug per kilogram of body weight). LD50 tests have been a feature of much of the testing of new drugs and cosmetics on animals prior to human exposure to those drugs and cosmetics. Animal-rights and animal–welfare groups have campaigned vigor-ously against LD50 testing because its immediate aim is to cause death to at least half of its animal-subjects and because many of those animals experience slow, painful dying.

Legalism: A term used in at least two different senses in the literature of bioethics. First, it can refer (usually pejora-tively) to a rather rigid adherence to moral principles and rules in one's moral judgments and choices, with little room for contextual evaluation or openness to possible exceptions. Second, it can refer to a tendency to address questions about the moral appropriateness of certain actions and practices by instead reframing those questions as matters of legal permissi-bility or impermissibility, thus essentially evading the process of genuine moral reflection.

Leukotomy (prefrontal lobotomy): A procedure first devel-oped in the early twentieth century that involves partial destruction of or severing of the neurological connections to and from the **frontal lobes** of the brain. First employed as a potential treatment for schizophrenia, depression, anxi-ety disorders, and various other mental afflictions, leukotomy also became infamous for its use as a means of "cure" for dis-ruptive behaviors, unpopular political ideologies, and homo-sexual behaviors. With the development of significant psy-choactive drugs beginning in the 1950s, the perceived need for leukotomy declined. It is rarely used today.

Linkage, genetic: The occurrence of two or more gene **alleles** (at different chromosome locations) being inherited jointly. Normally in **meiosis** each allele will be passed on ran-domly as new cells are created by cell division, but "genetic linkage" denotes the phenomenon in which particular alleles (especially some located on the same chromosome) are passed on together.

Living will: A form of advance directive, in document form, that allows its author to define the types of medical treatment that he would choose to receive, as well as those that would be unwanted (and under what conditions), in the event the author becomes unable to choose or communicate those treatment choices in the future. In other words, the living will is a form of prospective consent to, or rejection of, specified forms of treatment—quite often life-extending treatments. (See **advance directive**)

Lobotomy: See **leukotomy**

Locked-in syndrome: A rare neurological condition in which all voluntary muscles in the body are paralyzed except (usually) those controlling eye movement. Individuals with this disorder are fully conscious and can think, see, and hear but cannot move or speak. Communication may be possible though eye blinking. Locked-in syndrome may result from stroke or other brain trauma, drug overdose, or diseases that affect the sheath surrounding nerve cells. There is no cure or standard treatment for the condition, and the recovery of voluntary muscle function is rare.

$\backsim$ **M** $\backsim$

Macroallocation: Decisions to apportion or allocate resources (usually funding) for particular kinds of goods or services and determine the methods of their distribution. For instance, federal funding for Medicare, the Veteran's Administration (VA) hospital system, or the National Parks Service requires macroallocation decisions. (See **allocation**)

Magnetic resonance imaging (MRI): A technology using radio-frequency waves and a strong magnetic field to produce detailed images of internal organs and tissues. In this technology, radio-frequency waves cause intermittent excitement of hydrogen protons in a strong electromagnetic field. The radio signals emitted by the protons are computer-processed to form a three-dimensional image.

Malignant: Tending to be severe and to progress toward a more threatening state. Malignant tumors or cells, for instance, are those that invade and destroy neighboring tissues or spread (metastasize) to other parts of the body.

Malpractice: A type of legal tort in which, through malfeasance (wrongdoing), misfeasance (incorrect action), or nonfeasance (lack of appropriate action), a person who has a professional duty to act fails to follow accepted professional standards so as to cause injury to a person under her care or responsibility.

Managed care: In U.S. health care, organized techniques and systems employed to provide needed health care services while limiting or controlling their usage for purposes of cost efficiency. Typical managed care techniques include case management and review, review of proposed treatments for their medical necessity, and incentives to utilize particular health care providers and institutions—especially those whose reimbursement for services entails financial risk-sharing on their part. Perhaps the earliest large-scale application of managed care techniques occurred in the early 1980s with the U.S. government's alteration of the Medicare program to include fixed reimbursements through "diagnosis-related groups" (DRGs). In this program, hospitals would be reimbursed a fixed amount based upon a patient's diagnosis and projected plan of treatment, regardless of the hospital's actual costs in treating the patient. Over time, a variety of **managed care organizations (MCOs)** have been developed to provide care in a cost-efficient manner. The **health maintenance organization (HMO),** the earliest idea for managed care delivery, is a health insurance plan in which the insurer manages and controls all aspects of covered health care services for the insured person. Each insured person is assigned a primary care physician (PCP) responsible for providing needed health care overall, either personally or by providing specific referrals to specialist providers. Usually all services must be provided by physicians and other providers employed or contracted by the HMO, except in emergencies. In the majority of HMO arrangements, each insured is "capitated"—i.e., his primary care physician is paid a fixed amount for providing/referring all needed care within a given year. Also, most HMO arrangements require (usually small) copayments by the insured for each visit to a provider. In a **preferred provider organization (PPO),** a group of physicians, hospitals, and other providers contract with an insurer or administrator to provide health care services to their insured PPO members at a significant discount from their usual fees. Thus, in theory at least, providers get a steady stream of PPO-insured patients, the insurer can pay for needed care at a discount, and the insured should benefit from lower insurance premiums. **Point of service (POS)** plans, sometimes described as a hybrid of HMO and PPO plans, include a network of contracted care providers (from which, as in the HMO, the insured selects a primary care physician to coordinate her care). However, insured persons are free to select options for care outside the "managed" aspects of the system at a higher out-of-pocket cost to themselves. For instance, they may choose to seek care from an in-network specialist with a referral from their PCP and pay only a small copayment; or they may choose to seek care from a particular in-network specialist without a referral and pay a larger portion of the specialist's fee; or they may seek care from an out-of-network provider and pay a substantially larger portion of the provider's fee. Finally, in addition to these examples of managed care organizations, many insurers are also including aspects of managed care techniques in "traditional" or "indemnity" health insurance plans (i.e., plans in which the insured chooses the health provider and the insurer pays a certain percentage of the provider's "usual and customary" fees, subject to an annual deductible by the insured), especially such features as utilization reviews (of health care resources in the delivery of care) and the requirement of precertification for non-emergency hospital admissions.

Mature minor doctrine: In medico-legal contexts, the doctrine under which children (in the United States, persons younger than eighteen years) may be regarding as having the same right to give consent (for treatment, or for withholding or withdrawing treatment) as adult persons. The doctrine has found application, for instance, in circumstances where contraceptive and abortion services are sought by minor persons and in cases involving disagreements between a minor patient and his parent(s) regarding the acceptability of treatment(s) for that minor patient. Court decisions regarding possible recognition of mature minor status frequently cite a variety of factors to be weighed in making that judgment, including age; ability; experience; education; training; degree of maturity or judgment exhibited by the child; conduct or demeanor exhibited by the child in the decision-making context; and the child's apparent capacity to appreciate the nature, risks, and consequences of any medical procedure to be performed (or withheld). Some judicial opinions and state statutes immunize physicians from liability for failure to obtain parental consent for a minor's treatment or nontreatment (in cases where the child and his parent[s] disagree) based upon the physician's "good faith estimate" of the minor's maturity level. (See, e.g., Angela R. Holder, *Legal Issues in Pediatric and Adolescent Medicine,* 2nd ed. [New Haven: Yale University Press, 1985].)

MCO (managed care organization):   See **managed care**

Means and ends: Terms used in philosophical discourse to refer to the recognized goals, purposes or intended outcomes of human choices—that is, the "ends" being sought—and those courses of action selected to achieve or bring about those goals or outcomes—that is, the "means" to those "ends."

Meiosis: The process of cell division in sexually reproducing organisms in which the number of **chromosomes** is reduced from **diploid** (two of each type of chromosome, in pairs) to **haploid** (a set of single chromosomes). In animals, meiosis leads to the development of **gametes** (sperm and ova), which are chromosomally haploid.

Metaethics: The exploration and explanation of the meaning of moral concepts, moral language, and forms of moral reasoning. For example, metaethics may explore whether social morality is emotive or rational, objective, or subjective. Or it may examine the meaning of moral terms such as "value," "responsibility," "virtue," "principle," or "rights." It also includes the study of moral epistemology (i.e., theories of the sources and forms of moral knowledge) and forms or methods of moral reasoning and **justification.** (See **ethics**)

Metastasis: From Greek meaning "removal from one place to another"; the process in which cancer spreads from the place where it began to other, distant parts of the body. The term can also refer to the area of new cancer growth that has resulted from the movement of cancer cells or tissues from another part of the body.

MFPR: See **multifetus pregnancy reduction**

Microallocation: Decisions to apportion or allot among persons particular resources that are scarce either naturally or because of previous **macroallocation** decisions. Distribution of scarce cadaver organs for transplant among the many potential recipients is an example of microallocation. The term **"rationing"** is sometimes employed as a synonym for microallocation although some commentators also use that term to refer to certain macroallocation decisions as well. (See **allocation**)

Microinjection: The injection of **DNA** or other substance into a single living cell by means of a very fine micro needle. This procedure has been used, for example, in **genetic engineering** and in the production of **transgenic animals.**

Mifepristone (RU-486):   A synthetic steroid compound developed primarily for use as a contraceptive and **abortifacient.** In small doses it acts as a regular contraceptive, preventing ovulation. In somewhat larger doses it can act as an "emergency contraceptive" to prevent pregnancy after sexual intercourse. When used as an abortifacient (in the first two months of pregnancy) mifepristone blocks the effects of pregnancy hormones upon the lining of the uterus and, when combined with contraction-causing prostaglandin compounds, leads to chemically induced abortion.

Mitochondria (singular = mitochondrion):   Structures within the cytoplasm of cells but outside its nucleus that provide energy for the cell. Mitochondria also include a portion of **DNA** (in humans, each mitochondrion contains the DNA for thirty-seven **genes**), which can influence the development of an organism in addition to the genetic pattern determined by its chromosomal DNA.

Mongolism: A term once used to refer to **Down syndrome,** or Trisomy 21. (See **aneuploidy**)

Monogenic disorder: A genetic condition or disorder caused by the deletion, mutation, or replacement of a single **gene.**

Monosomy: A genetic condition in which one chromosome of a matched pair of chromosomes is absent. (See **aneuploidy**)

Monozygotic twin: One of a pair of individuals developed from a single fertilized ovum (zygote) that has divided into two separate collections of cells early in the process of development. Monozygotic twins are often referred to as "identical twins." (See **twins**)

Moral relativism: See **relativism, moral**

Morbidity: A term generally referring to the state of being diseased or unhealthy but that can also refer to the relative prevalence, incidence, or severity of disease within a given community or population.

Mortality: Broadly, the quality of being mortal and subject to death. The term can also refer, however, to the rate of deaths within a given population or to the ratio of expected deaths to actual deaths.

Morula: The solid mass of cells (**blastomeres**) resulting from the splitting of the fertilized egg (**zygote**) in the earliest stages of **embryonic development.**

MRI: See **magnetic resonance imaging**

Multifactorial disorder: See **polygenic disorder**

Multifetal pregnancy reduction (MFPR):   A form of **abortion** in which one or more fetuses in a multifetal pregnancy are selectively aborted to allow for more enhanced development and viability of the remaining fetus or fetuses, and to prevent miscarriage or very premature delivery for the remaining fetus or fetuses. This procedure is usually performed between weeks 10 and 12 of pregnancy, and most commonly reduces the number of fetuses to two. Broadened usage of **assisted**

reproductive technologies and fertility drugs in recent years have led to dramatic increases in the incidence of "high order" pregnancies [with three or more fetuses]. Risks of miscarriage, stillbirth, and permanent disabilities increase with each additional fetus beyond two; thus the MFPR procedure attempts to minimize those risks for some fetuses by reducing the number of fetuses developing together in the uterus.

Multiple pregnancy: A pregnancy involving two or more fetuses.

Multipotency: The capacity of a cell to divide and develop into more than one type or line of cells. (See **stem cells**)

Mutagen: An agent or substance that causes genetic **mutation.**

Mutagenesis: The process of inducing genetic **mutation.**

Mutation, genetic: A change in genetic material (such as a strand of **DNA**) that is transmitted to the next generations of an organism's cells through cell division and replication.

‿N‿

Nasogastric tube: A form of **feeding tube** used to deliver nutrition, hydration, or medications to the stomach of a patient who is unable to consume them in the normal manner. The nasogastric tube is a flexible tube that is introduced through the nasal passageway into the esophagus and down into the stomach. Usually nasogastric tubes are used only on a temporary basis and not for long-term nutritional support of persons unable to eat or drink. (See also **PEG tube**)

Natural family planning (NFP):   Term used to describe several methods for timing or preventing conception and pregnancy that do not employ chemical or other "artificial" means of contraception (and which are therefore generally accepted by the hierarchy of the Roman Catholic Church). One type of NFP involves periodic abstinence from sexual activity during the fertile periods of a woman's menstrual cycle. This may be accomplished via "observational" methods, in which certain biological signs or indicators of fertility are used as guides for when sexual abstinence is indicated; or via "statistical" or "calendar" methods, in which the probability of fertile/infertile periods of the menstrual cycle are inferred based upon the length of previous menstrual cycles. A form of this latter method is often referred to as the **rhythm method.** The other major type of NFP, the "lactational amenorrhea method," relies upon the natural suspension of menstrual cycles occurring during the breastfeeding of infants. (A strict version of this method is known as "ecological breastfeeding.")

Naturalistic fallacy: Philosopher G. E. Moore's claim (in his *Principia Ethica*, 1903) of logical fallacy on the part of those who seek to justify their moral conclusions by defining that which is intrinsically "good" in terms of natural properties such as biological survivability, evolutionary development, or pleasure. Since Moore's original arguments, the term has also been used to refer more broadly to the "is–ought problem," that is, the (claimed) logical fallacy of deriving conclusions about what one *ought* to do from observations about what *is* in the observed processes, structures, or tendencies of the natural world. Some have argued, for example, contrary to the assertions of some forms of traditional **natural law** ethics, that claims about what human beings ought to do cannot be derived from observations about the "natural" tendencies or inclinations (e.g., to prolong one's life, to mate and reproduce) of humans and other living things.

Natural law: In ethical theory, the concept of a set of norms or "laws" observable by human reason in (or inferred from) the patterns and functions of nature (including human nature) and providing objective, universal guidance for human moral choices. In Western philosophical history, Socrates, Plato, and Aristotle all emphasized distinctions between what might be recognized as "natural justice" or "natural right," applicable at all times and in all places, as compared with notions of justice or right from social convention or custom. The most prominent contemporary version of natural law theory is that of the Roman Catholic Church. Many early Christian thinkers sought to incorporate natural law concepts, especially Aristotelian and Stoic ideas, into their theological projects. The most influential Christian natural law thinker, Thomas Aquinas (1225–1274), posited a vast, multilayered, and interconnected theory of "law." In

Thomas's system the *eternal law* (which exists only in the mind of God) orders and governs all the cosmos; the *natural law* is that part of the eternal law which can be apprehended by unaided human reason; the *divine law* is that aspect of the eternal law made known to humanity through divine revelation; and *human law* is the practical reason's application of the precepts of natural law to the particular conditions or situations of human life in community (thus, any legitimate human law [or moral choice] must be consistent with the precepts of natural law). (See his *Summa Theologiae* I-II, qq. 90–95.) In this general framework, the moral rightness of any action is a function of whether that action is directed to (or at least does not deny) its proper natural end or purpose (toward which we can rationally perceive a "natural inclination"). One well-known contemporary example of this kind of natural law reasoning is represented in recent papal denunciations of artificial contraception (by Pius XI, Paul VI, and John Paul II, for example). The problem with artificial contraception in this view is that its employment in conjunction with sexual intercourse directly and intentionally frustrates (or fails to be "open to") the proper "natural" end or purpose of the sex organs and sex drive—namely, the procreation and rearing of offspring. On the other hand, **natural family planning** may be acceptable in some cases because, although it does entail at least temporary contraceptive intent, its practice remains very much open to the possibility of conception and thus it does not frustrate the natural purpose of sexual intercourse. Contemporary Catholic debates about natural law theory center around concerns such as whether moral rules derived from natural law are absolute and without exception; whether traditional interpretations of what reason discerns from "nature" have been too rigid and inflexible, too physical-descriptive (as opposed to contextual and personal), and too "classicist" in form; whether one good or value identified through natural law may ever be sacrificed directly, or only indirectly, for the sake of preserving another value; and so on. (See, e.g., Charles E. Curran and Richard A. McCormick, eds., *Readings in Moral Theology No. 7: Natural Law and Theology,* [New York: Paulist Press, 1991].) (See also **double effect, rule or principle of;** and **totality, principle of**)

Naturopathy: A form of health care, with roots in nineteenth-century Europe (especially Germany) that emphasizes support of health rather than the combating of disease. Among the central beliefs of naturopathy are that nature has a healing power and that living organisms have the power to maintain or regain a state of balance and health. In assisting the body's attempts to regain health, naturopathic practitioners tend to employ means they consider most natural and least invasive. Typical forms of naturopathic management or treatment may include dietary changes and dietary supplements, herbal medicines, hydrotherapy, exercise therapy, physical manipulations and mobilization techniques, or mind–body therapies such as meditation and yoga. Naturopathy is generally considered a form of "complementary and alternative" medicine as opposed to "conventional" medicine. However, naturopathic physicians may receive training in several four-year graduate-level naturopathic medical schools in the United States, and seventeen states and territories have laws regulating licensure and the practice of naturopathy.

Negative eugenics: Programs and policies designed to discourage or prevent reproduction by those deemed to be genetically unhealthy or "unfit" (i.e., those seen to be carriers of negative traits or conditions that might be inherited by any of their offspring). (See **eugenics**)

Neomort: A term meaning "newly dead." In a 1974 article by Willard Gaylin, the term was specifically applied to individuals who meet criteria for the determination of **brain death** but who, with technological life support in place, continue to respire, circulate blood, digest, excrete, and so on. Gaylin posed questions about how such individuals should be treated in light of their obvious usefulness as teaching and experimentation subjects, preservation/storage units for transplantable organs and tissues, and so on.

Neonatology: The study, diagnosis, and treatment of disorders occurring in newborn infants.

Neoplasm: A tumor or other new and abnormal cell or tissue growth, specifically when cell growth is progressive and uncontrolled. Neoplasms may be malignant or benign.

Neural tube defect: A defect involving the brain or spinal cord that occurs during **embryonic development.** In the embryo, the precursor of what will become the central nervous system is the neural groove, which develops and closes to form the neural tube, which develops further to become the spinal cord and brain. Neural tube defects represent "mistakes" in that developmental process. Examples of these defects include **anencephaly** (a condition caused by failure of the forward end of the neural tube to fully close, so that the infant is born without a forebrain [or cerebral hemispheres] and with remaining brain tissue often not covered by skull or skin), **hydranencephaly** (in which the cerebral hemispheres are absent, and replaced by sacs of cerebrospinal fluid), **spina bifida** (in which the spinal cord does not develop fully and protrudes between also-undeveloped vertebrae), and **encephalocele** (in which one or more plates in the developing skull fail to seal, so that brain tissue and its membrane covering protrude through the gap in the skull).

Neurotoxin: A chemical or other substance that exerts a poisonous or destructive effect on tissues in the nervous system (e.g., nerve, spinal cord, or brain tissues).

NFP: See **natural family planning**

Non-heart-beating donor (NHBD):   A person who is allowed to experience cessation of heartbeat and respiration after removal of life-support technology, after which organs or tissues are surgically removed for transplant purposes. (See **donation after cardiac death**)

Nonmaleficence: The refraining from inflicting harm upon others. In the history of Western Hippocratic medicine, the duty of nonmaleficence has found popular expression in the maxim **primum non nocere** ("first, or above all, do no harm"), widely considered to be the most fundamental moral obligation of health care. The moral principle of nonmaleficence entails a negative obligation—to not inflict harm—that is often seen as the complementary converse of the obligation entailed by the principle of **beneficence**—to do good for the other. There has been considerable debate about where the negative duty of nonmaleficence ends and the positive duty of beneficence begins, especially because the former duty has been regarded in most Western societies (at least since the Enlightenment) as prior or more clearly obligatory. For example, are the duties to avoid or prevent the creation of harmful conditions, to warn others of the existence of risks of harm, or to remove harmful conditions before they can have effect, to be considered basic duties of nonmaleficence or perhaps more ideal (and less obligatory) charitable acts of beneficence? (See, e.g., Tom L. Beauchamp and James F. Childress, *Principles of Biomedical Ethics,* 6th ed. [New York: Oxford University Press, 2009], chapter 5.)

Nonreproductive cloning: Cloning procedures undertaken to produce early **embryos** whose **stem cells** can be harvested for medical research and therapeutic purposes. (See **cloning**)

Nontherapeutic research: Medical experimentation usually involving healthy volunteer subjects instead of sick persons because it is concerned solely with yielding experimental data and is not aimed at providing any therapy for the subjects. (See **experimentation, medical**)

Normative ethics: Ethical theories that attempt to identify those moral norms, values, or traits that should be accepted as standards or guides for moral behavior and moral judgments. (See **ethics**)

Nucleotides: Chemical compounds that are the structural units of **DNA, RNA,** and several chemical cofactors in cell metabolism.

Nucleus, cell: In cell biology the membrane-enclosed part of the cell containing most of the cell's genetic material arranged as long **DNA** and protein strands that form **chromosomes.**

Nuremberg Code: Name given to a set of moral principles for the conduct of medical **experimentation** involving human subjects, delivered by judges in the trials of so-called Nazi doctors at Nuremburg, Germany, following World War II (1947). Defendants in these "doctors' trials" had been charged with performing gruesome (often fatal) experiments upon nonconsenting persons, mostly concentration camp inmates. While they were formally charged with experimentation without the consent of their subjects, they were essentially being charged with "crimes against humanity." In their defense, however, many of the accused physicians argued that there were no existing laws defining legal and illegal forms of experimentation. Thus, along with delivering their judicial verdicts, the Nuremburg judges presented ten principles that, in their view, were necessary for any experiment involving human subjects to be legally and morally acceptable. The first of these ten principles established the absolute necessity of the voluntary, uncoerced **informed consent** of any potential research subject. Other principles addressed the demands of **beneficence, nonmaleficence,** and proper scientific formulation in any human experimentation. The Nuremburg Code was adopted almost immediately as a set of moral guidelines for experimentation by the American Medical Association (although numerous examples of violations of the code in U.S. medical research have come to light in recent decades). Parts of the Nuremburg Code have been incorporated into federal regulations governing research in institutions receiving federal funding and have been incorporated into the laws of some countries and U.S. states (such as California).

O

Oligospermia: A condition in which the male testes produce very few **spermatozoa** (sperm cells). As a clinical measure, oligospermia is diagnosed when an ejaculate of semen contains less than 20 million spermatozoa per milliliter.

Oncogene: A modified **gene** or **DNA** segment that codes for a protein believed to cause cancer. Oncogenes may be activated by genetic **mutations,** and their activation increases the chance that a normal cell will develop into a tumor cell. In many cases a viral gene will cause this transformation of normal to tumor cell.

Oncology: The medical specialty that studies tumors (cancers) and their prevention, development, diagnosis, and treatment.

Ontogeny: The entire developmental history of an individual organism. Thus, the ontogeny of a human individual would encompass all stages of **embryonic development,** birth, infancy, adolescence, adulthood, and old age.

Oocyte: An immature **ovum** (egg cell).

Oophorectomy: Surgical removal of the female ovary or ovaries.

Orchiectomy: Surgical removal of the male testis or testes (castration).

Organizational ethics (in health care): Term used to denote moral reflection and analysis regarding decisions and actions taken by health care organizations and institutions (e.g., by administrators, institutional board and committee members, and others with institutional authority). Organizational ethics has its roots in the discipline of business ethics, and it is often contrasted popularly with "clinical ethics" (the former relating to the "business" side of health care ethics, and the latter to the "patient care" side). However, in the practice of health care delivery, such a distinction is neither neat nor simple. A major incentive for focus upon organizational ethics in the United States came from the Joint Commission on the Accreditation of Health Care Organizations (**JCAHO**), whose 1995 Accreditation Standards first included requirements regarding what was termed "organization ethics." These standards mandated that health care institutions have codes of ethical behavior regarding patient admissions, transfer, discharge and billing practices, marketing practices, and relationships of the institution and its staff with other health care providers, educational institutions, and payers. Furthermore, institutions were required to have in place policies and procedures to protect the integrity of clinical decision making regardless of the financial arrangements available to compensate recommended treatments. As concerns for the practice and promotion of organizational ethics have expanded over the past few decades, some health care institutions have established new **institutional ethics committees (IEC)** dedicated to the consideration of organizational ethics issues in particular; others have combined a focus on organizational ethics along with clinical ethics in a single IEC structure. Common organizational ethics concerns faced by most health care institutions include employee relations and the provision of just wages, benefits, and working conditions; discrimination practices toward (or by) employees; protections for confidentiality of patient information; provision of uncompensated care for poor and uninsured persons; restrictions or limitations imposed by **managed care** arrangements; and environmental impacts within the community.

Organ transplantation: See **transplantation, organ and tissue**

Ovarian follicle: See **follicle, ovarian**

Ovum: An egg cell; the female **gamete,** or germ cell.

ᔜ **P** ᔛ

Palliative care: Medical care or treatment that is focused upon ameliorating the symptoms (e.g., pain, discomfort, depression) of a disease or condition rather than being curative. In **hospice** care, the aim of palliative care is to provide comfort and well-being rather than to prolong life.

Pantheism: The view that the divine is in everything that exists, or that all of nature and the universe is equivalent to an immanent, abstract, all-encompassing God. This essential identification of the existent universe with "God" stands in contrast to the view of *panentheism* that God exists beyond and outside the universe but interpenetrates all parts of nature.

Paraplegia: Paralysis (loss of motor function) in the legs and lower part of the body.

Parthenogenesis: A form of asexual reproduction in which an embryo or seed develops without **fertilization** by a male organism. While common in some plant and non-mammalian animal species, parthenogenesis is rare in animal species that have X and Y sex chromosomes. However, unfertilized human and other mammalian ova (eggs) may spontaneously activate and begin to divide; they may also be deliberately stimulated, chemically or electrically, to begin that process. While parthenogenesis has been used to produce a fatherless mouse, as yet there are no reported cases of parthenogenetic reproduction in humans. The process has, however, been used to stimulate unfertilized human ova to divide and develop to the **blastocyst** stage of **embryonic development**—the stage at which **stem cells** may be harvested from the developing embryo.

Partial-birth abortion (dilation and extraction):   A controversial surgical abortion procedure involving cervical dilation followed by partial delivery of the intact fetus feet first; then a sharp instrument is inserted into the back of the fetus's head and the brain is suctioned before delivery is completed. (See **abortion**)

Passive euthanasia: A form of "letting die" or "allowed death" in which death is intentionally brought about by withholding or withdrawing some form of treatment that could otherwise sustain life. (See **euthanasia**)

Paternalism: Actions taken toward another person without their consent, or a refusal to accept that person's own choices, desires, or actions, intended solely for the benefit of that person. Some commentators distinguish between "weak" or "limited" paternalism and "strong" or "extended" paternalism. In weak or limited paternalism, the paternalist attempts to benefit, or prevent self-harming choices by, another person who is also perceived to be incompetent or otherwise incapable of rational, knowledgeable, willing, choosing, or acting for herself. In "strong" or "extended" paternalism, the paternalist attempts to benefit, or prevent self-harming choices by, another person who is fully competent to make his own self-regarding choices.

Pathogen: Any substance or microorganism that causes disease or illness in its host organism.

Patient Self-Determination Act (PSDA):   Federal legislation enacted (as an amendment to the Omnibus Budget Reconciliation Act of 1990) with the intent of protecting and promoting individual **autonomy** and **self-determination** regarding health care treatment choices for individuals. The act establishes obligations for health care institutions that receive federal funding (hospitals, nursing homes, retirement facilities, home health agencies, and many managed care organizations) to provide education and assistance to their patients, clients, or residents regarding their health care decision-making rights and their opportunities to create **advance directives** for health care in accordance with law in each state. Institutions are also charged to similarly educate their staff members and members of surrounding communities, and are prohibited from discriminating against persons who do not have (or do not want) advance directives.

PEG tube: Percutaneous endoscopic gastrostomy tube, a form of **"feeding tube"** used to deliver nutrition, hydration, or medications to the stomach of a patient who is unable to consume them normally. Generally, the PEG tube is preferred for long-term artificial provision of nutrition or hydration, whereas temporary or short-term provision may be accomplished via the **nasogastric tube.** The PEG tube is inserted via a small incision through the skin, abdominal wall, and the wall of the stomach. Placement of the tube in the stomach is guided by an endoscope (a long flexible tube with a light source and camera lens at its end) inserted through the mouth and down the esophagus into the stomach. Liquid nourishment and medications can then be introduced into the interior of the stomach via the end of the PEG tube extending outside the abdomen.

Peripherally inserted central catheter (PICC):   An intravenous catheter used to inject fluids, nutrition, or medications into the bloodstream when such injection cannot be accomplished safely or efficiently via a routine peripheral IV (intravenous) site. The PICC is inserted into a peripheral vein (usually in the arm) and then guided through successively larger veins into the superior vena cava (a large vein leading into the heart). With the tip of the catheter opening into this major vein with rapid, high-volume flow of blood, it is possible to deliver fluids and chemicals in quantities and concentrations that would be toxic, irritating, or overwhelming if delivered into a smaller, more peripheral vein. Thus the PICC can be useful for the delivery of long or concentrated chemotherapy regimens, extended antibiotic therapies, and hyperalimentation or total peripheral nutrition.

Persistent vegetative state (PVS):   A state of prolonged unconsciousness and unawareness, sometimes following **coma,** in which the individual has lost higher brain functions (such as thinking ability and awareness of surroundings) but maintains basic functions such as breathing, heart regulation, and normal sleep cycles. Persons in PVS may exhibit spontaneous movements or responses such as grimaces, laughs, cries, or eye-opening, either randomly or in response to external stimuli (especially loud or painful stimuli). According to some authorities, a "vegetative state" becomes a "persistent vegetative state" only if it persists for more than thirty days. However, many in the neurological community insist on a more complex distinction between "vegetative state," "continuing vegetative state," and "permanent vegetative state."

Personhood: In the discourse of ethics, a term that usually refers to the moral status of an individual as an agent or person not only genetically human and biologically alive but as also bearing the moral rights and obligations of membership in the human community. There is much controversy, of course, regarding the criterion (or set of criteria) that defines the beginning (and end) of human personhood. Some argue that the inheritance of human genes from two human parents to create a new and unique human entity marks the arrival of personhood; thus a person would be a person from the moment of **conception** or **fertilization**. Others, such as philosophers Mary Anne Warren and Peter Singer and theologian Joseph Fletcher, have argued for sets of criteria (e.g., consciousness, reasoning, self-awareness) that must be met developmentally before a living, genetically human fetus or infant might be regarded as having personhood. In American legal history, live birth has been the point at which legal personhood, including the rights and protections of citizenship, has been recognized (although some states have laws that punish harms done to fetuses prebirth in a manner equivalent to punishments for harms to persons already born). In contemporary American society, the ongoing and heated debate about how to answer the question "When does life begin?" is in reality a debate about the point at which moral (and legal) personhood should or must be recognized and respected.

PET scan: See **positron emission tomography**

PGD: See **preimplantation genetic diagnosis**

Pharmaceutical formulary: See **formulary, pharmaceutical**

Pharmacodynamics: The study of the physiological and biochemical effects of drugs upon the body, the mechanisms of action of drugs within the body, and the relationship between the concentration of the drug and its effects upon the body.

Pharmacogenetics: The study of genetic variation among (usually one or a few) genes that causes a differing response to drugs by an organism. A related area of study, pharmacogenomics, applies **genomic** technologies to improving the applications of existing drugs and the development of new and more effective drugs by identifying genetic determinants in an organism's responses to drugs.

Pharmacokinetics: Study of what happens to substances (e.g., drugs) introduced into the body in terms of their absorption by the body, their distribution throughout the body, their metabolism by the body into other compounds or byproducts, and the excretion of those metabolic results by the body.

Phenotype: The outward, observable expression of physical traits that are variable among individuals. The term can refer to the overall physical appearance and constitution of the individual or to a specific manifestation of a particular trait (such as eye color). Phenotype is determined in part by **genotype** (the genetic constitution of the individual) as well as by environmental factors and by random variation in the phenotypic expression of some genotypes. One simple expression of this is genotype + environment + random selection = phenotype.

Physician-assisted suicide (PAS):   See **suicide**

PICC (or PIC line):   See **peripherally inserted central catheter**

Pittsburgh Protocol: A policy developed at the University of Pittsburgh Hospitals in the early 1990s for harvesting transplantable organs from persons who have not experienced **brain death** but are instead **"non-heart-beating donors" (NHBD)**

due to cessation of spontaneous breathing and heartbeat. (See **donation after cardiac death**)

Placebo: In health care practice, a substance or procedure applied to the body that has no recognized physiological or therapeutic effect but which is used to promote a therapeutic or palliative effect (the "placebo effect") by causing the recipient to believe that it is a physiologically active substance. In randomized medical **experimentation** projects involving the comparative testing of one form of treatment against no treatment, the placebo is the inactive substance given to the subjects in the "control" or nontreatment arm of the experiment in such a way that all subjects, or researchers and subjects, are unaware of which subjects are receiving experimental treatment or placebo.

Pleasure principle: See **utilitarianism**

Pluripotency: In biology, the capacity of a cell to divide and give rise to most, but not all, of the cell and tissue types necessary for the development of a complete organism. For example, embryonic **stem cells** taken from a human **blastocyst** are pluripotent in that they can give rise to all three embryonic germ layers and thus to all internal human tissues, but they cannot give rise to the extraembryonic tissues (e.g., the placenta).

Point of service (POS): A form of **managed care organization (MCO)** for the provision of health insurance. (See **managed care**)

Polygenic disorder: A genetic disorder resulting from the effects of multiple genes or from gene expression in combination with environmental and lifestyle factors. (See **disorder, genetic**)

Polymerase: An **enzyme** active in the process of cell division and multiplication by enabling the formation of new, complementary strands of **DNA** and **RNA** to join with each of the single strands resulting after the splitting of the double-stranded DNA/RNA.

Polymorphism: In biological terms, common, natural variations of a **gene, DNA** sequence, or **chromosome** resulting in multiple **alleles** of a gene within a population, usually producing multiple **phenotypes** for the same genetic characteristic.

Polyploid: Having more than two of each set of chromosomes in the cell nucleus of an organism. (See **aneuploidy**)

POS: See **point of service**

Positive eugenics: Programs established to encourage and enable the maximal level of reproduction by those deemed to be most genetically "fit" or who bear the most socially desirable heritable traits. (See **eugenics**)

Positron emission tomography (PET):   A form of diagnostic scan that can produce images of body organs and tissues by detecting positrons (tiny particles emitted by radioactive substances injected into the body). PET scans are often used to detect tumors and cancer cells (and changes to them produced by chemotherapy) as well as adequacy of blood flow to the heart and other organs and tissues, etc.

Posthumous gamete donation: Extraction of sperm (or ova) from the body of a person declared clinically dead (generally, brain dead), most often to accomplish procreation by that person (using assisted reproductive technology) posthumously, at the request of a spouse or partner.

PPO (preferred provider organization):   See **managed care**

Preconception injury: In tort law, the claim of damage to a child in pregnancy or after birth caused by the harmful or negligent action of another person toward that child's mother (or father) before the child was conceived. For example, a mother might seek damages against the manufacturer of birth control pills she had been taking by claiming the pills were defective and caused chromosomal damage to the child she later conceived.

Preembryo (or proembryo):   Term used to describe the stage of cell development from the point of **fertilization** of the ovum by sperm until the **implantation** of the **blastocyst** into the lining of the uterus.

Prefrontal cortex: The anterior (forward) part of the **frontal lobes** of the brain. This area is responsible for what is called "executive function"—i.e., coordination of thoughts and actions with internal goals. Executive function includes the capacity to plan and work toward defined goals, recognize similarities and differences, distinguish between good and bad or better and best, predict outcomes of one's actions, and suppress urges that could lead to actions understood to be socially or legally unacceptable.

Prefrontal lobotomy: See **leukotomy**

Pregnancy reduction: See **multifetal pregnancy reduction**

Preimplantation genetic diagnosis (PGD):   A technique involving both genetic diagnostic technology and **assisted reproductive technology** to gain genetic information about a newly conceived embryo prior to the establishment of uterine pregnancy. Following **in vitro fertilization,** one or two cells may be split off from the developing **morula** (see **embryonic development**) and subjected to genetic testing to diagnose sex, chromosomal constitution (**karyotype**), and genes or gene markers for known genetic diseases or disorders. Diagnostic information obtained in this way may then be used by parents to determine which (or whether) tested embryos will be transferred to the mother's uterus for implantation, pregnancy, and birth. PGD was originally developed to allow carriers of serious x-linked genetic disorders to select only female embryos for implantation. Moral debate has arisen regarding the use of PGD to "screen out" embryos with much less serious conditions, or embryos whose sex is not the sex preferred by the parents at this point. Some critics charge that the practice of PGD for genetic disease screening purposes is simply a new, high-tech expression of **eugenics;** that its use for sex selection (which is illegal in several countries) could lead to or exacerbate patterns of gender discrimination; and that it may lead parents to place unreasonable expectations upon children intentionally "selected" in this way.

Premarital testing (genetic):   Testing of couples to detect abnormal or disease-causing genetic conditions that may be inherited by future children, conducted prior to (and in some circumstances as a legal condition of) marriage.

Prenatal diagnosis: The use of diagnostic techniques to assess the health and condition of the developing fetus during pregnancy.

Prenatal genetic screening: The use of genetic diagnostic technologies to determine the genetic complement (as well as sex, chromosomal abnormalities, defective genes, etc.) of an embryo or fetus prior to birth.

Prescriptive ethics (normative ethics): See **ethics**

Presumed consent: Generally, a substitute for an individual's express **informed consent** that amounts to an assumption of consent inferred from his past willingness to give similar consents (or, more often, his lack of specific unwillingness to consent). For example, several countries have public policies of "presumed consent" for the donation of individuals' organs after death. Consent is presumed unless the individual has made objection (oral, written, or via national "nondonor" computer registry) to the postmortem retrieval of his organs. "Implied consent" and "tacit consent" are terms often considered synonymous with "presumed consent" although policies regulating the latter are sometimes accused of basing their standard of "presumption" on something other than what is actually implied by individuals' past behaviors.

Presymptomatic (or predictive) genetic testing: Testing used to detect gene **mutations** associated with diseases or disorders that occur after birth (or late in life) before symptoms of those diseases or disorders appear.

Primordial germ cells: Cells that exist in the embryo only early in the process of **embryonic development** but are precursors to what will become sperm and ova cells. Unlike mature germ cells, primordial germ cells are **diploid** in their chromosomal complement. However, as they associate closely with the **somatic cells** of the part of the embryo that will form **gonads** (testes and ovaries) they become irreversibly committed to development as **haploid** germ cells.

Primum non nocere: Latin phrase meaning "first [or above all] do no harm," which has been popularized in many Western health care contexts as the most fundamental principle of medical ethics from the Hippocratic tradition. The actual source of the phrase is not clear because it does not appear in any of the known writings of the Hippocratic Corpus. It does, however, clearly assert a duty of **nonmaleficence** that, when coupled with a duty of **beneficence** toward those seeking health care, is clearly asserted in the Hippocratic oath: "I will prescribe regimens for the good of my patients according to my ability and my judgment and never do harm to anyone."

Principle of totality: See **totality, principle of**

Prion: An infectious particle comprised of protein but unlike bacteria or viruses in that it is apparently lacking any complement of nucleic acid (**DNA** or **RNA**). Thus it is not susceptible to the types of antibacterial or antiviral treatments that modify or interfere with nucleic acids. Furthermore, prion diseases can develop as a result of infection and can be genetically inherited. Examples of prion diseases include bovine spongiform encephalopathy ("mad cow disease") and Creutzfeld-Jacob disease in humans. All known prion diseases affect the structure of the brain and other neural tissues and are not treatable.

Privilege, therapeutic: See **therapeutic privilege**

Procreation: The begetting of offspring by organisms via sexual **reproduction.**

Proportionalism: Beginning in the 1960s, a method of reasoning about the moral rightness or wrongness of actions developed by numerous "revisionist" Roman Catholic moral theologians such as Louis Janssens, Josef Fuchs, Peter Knauer,

Bruno Schuller, and Richard McCormick. The best-known and most controversial aspect of proportionalism is its rejection of some traditional Church teachings based in **natural law** reasoning that certain actions (usually related to biological processes or sexuality) are "intrinsic moral evils" regardless of the particular context or circumstances surrounding their performance. So, for example, recent Church teachings have held that use of artificial contraception is always intrinsically morally evil because it deliberately frustrates the possibility of sexual intercourse serving its natural good or purpose—the procreation and education of offspring. (Yet, these teachings have also held that **natural family planning** methods may be morally licit, even with deliberate contraceptive intent, because the means used does not disallow the biological possibility of conception.) The "proportionalist" response would be that the act of using artificial contraception, in and of itself, cannot yet be said to be a *moral* evil; it is rather a "premoral" (or "ontic," or "physical," or "nonmoral") evil—an act that would be morally evil unless there exists a "proportionate reason" for its performance as a means to a higher or more attainable value. Discernment of proportionate reason would require reflection concerning all values actually at stake in the situation—not only procreative potential but also mutual affirmation of love and faithfulness, health and well-being of parties involved, economic and social flourishing of the family, etc. Thus, moral discernment regarding proportionate reason would have to consider such questions as, "Does a choice for artificial contraception *in this circumstance* actually represent a permanent or ongoing rejection of procreative commitment?" "Would potential pregnancy *in this situation* constitute a risk to the values of physical, spiritual or emotional health, economic stability, or family unity?" "If expansion of family size is imprudent or even dangerous at this time, then is sacrifice of the value of mutual expression of love also inherently necessary?" and so on. Proportionalists argue that their approach is an attempt to "update" the natural law methodology already employed in most official Catholic moral teachings by removing a relatively small category of actions considered always morally evil in light of the fact that Church teachings have already been able to find "proportionate reason" to justify many other "premoral" evils such as killing, telling an untruth, mutilating a body, violating a promise, and so on. Many of their arguments are developed within discussions of the traditional rule or principle of the **double effect.** Supporters of proportionalism see it as an alternative to both the "physicalist" rigidity of much traditional natural law reasoning, on the one hand, and a **consequentialist** or **situation ethics** justification of acts based solely upon calculation of potential effects, on the other. Richard McCormick, SJ, the best-known American proponent of proportionalism, has suggested several criteria that must be met in determining whether proportionate reason exists for any given act: the means employed (i.e., the action itself) will not cause more harm than necessary to achieve the intended value; no other less harmful means exists in this circumstance to protect the value at stake; and the means (action) employed to realize or promote that value will not actually undermine the value. (See, e.g., Richard M. Gula, *Reason Informed by Faith: Foundations of Catholic Morality* [New York: Paulist Press, 1989], especially chapter 18; Charles E. Curran and Richard A. McCormick, SJ, eds., *Readings in Moral Theology No. 1: Moral Norms and Catholic Tradition* [New York: Paulist Press, 1979]; and Christopher Kaczor, ed., *Proportionalism: For and Against* [Milwaukee: Marquette University Press, 2000].)

Proprietary health facilities: For-profit health care institutions operated by private corporations or groups.

Proteomics: The large-scale study of the structure and function of proteins in living organisms. The term "proteomics" is intended to be analogous to **"genomics"**: while the latter is the study of the gene complement and functions in organisms, the former is the study of their protein complement and functions.

Protocol, research: In medical research, a document describing the purpose and potential benefits (and risks) of the experiment; the hypothesis or hypotheses to be tested or confirmed; the research methodology, materials, and procedures to be used; the **informed consent** process to be used with subjects; and considerations regarding statistical analysis.

Protoplasm: In biology, the living substance within the cell(s) of the organism. The content of the cell nucleus is known as *nucleoplasm*, and the other substances inside the cell belong to its *cytoplasm*.

Proxy consent: A replacement or substitution for genuine **informed consent** in which consent for the treatment or research participation of an individual who is incompetent or incapable of giving her own consent is given by another person acting as the patient/research subject's "proxy." Morally central to the notion of proxy consent is the condition that the proxy consenter ought to determine what the patient/subject *would* decide if she were able, or what would be in the best interests of that individual in the case of children or others who have no decisional history from which to infer a preference. (See **surrogate consent**)

PSDA: See **Patient Self-Determination Act**

Psychiatric will: A concept first proposed by psychiatrist (and critic of psychiatry) Thomas Szasz in the early 1980s, which would allow a competent, mentally stable individual to express prospective consents for psychiatric interventions in the event he should become mentally unstable and incompetent. In Szasz's view, this would be a form of **advance directive** for psychiatric care. Those who greatly fear the prospect of psychosis and have great confidence in psychiatric interventions could execute a "will" prospectively consenting to their own involuntary institutionalization and other psychiatric interventions in the future. Conversely, those who dread the power of psychiatry and wish to be protected from it would have a legal vehicle for recording their competent nonconsent to future psychiatric interventions regardless of their future incompetence and the "need" for treatment perceived by psychiatric professionals at that later time.

Psychosurgery: Surgery performed to alter or disable structures of the brain to modify cognition as a treatment for serious mental illness. A well-known historical example of psychosurgery is **leukotomy** (or prefrontal lobotomy), which has now been largely replaced by a somewhat less invasive procedure, bilateral cingulotomy. Other modern methods of psychosurgery involve destruction of parts of the brain with radiation (via the "gamma knife") and electrical stimulation of parts of the brain using **deep brain stimulation.**

PVS: See **persistent vegetative state**

∽Q∽

QALYs: See **quality-adjusted life years**

Quadriplegia: Paralysis (loss of motor function) in all four limbs.

Quality-adjusted life years (QALYs): In health care economics, a construct used to measure the quality and quantity of life anticipated to result from a given medical treatment or intervention. In addition to the number of years the intervention is expected to add to the person's life, a value is assigned to the "quality" of those years. So, for example, each year of perfect health would be assigned a value of 1.0, but years of life with increasingly severe health problems would be assigned progressively lower values, with death having a value of 0.0. QALYs are often assessed and cited in decisions regarding how to allocate (scarce) available health care resources among multiple medical treatment options.

Quality of life: A phrase that, used in its broadest sense, refers to an assessment of those economic, social, physical, and psychological conditions or possibilities that make life pleasant and "livable" (such as economic standard of living, health, happiness, aesthetic experiences, freedom, opportunities for innovation). In health care contexts, however, references to "quality of life" are most often made in circumstances involving incompetent persons (who cannot make known their own degree of satisfaction with their life conditions) for whom decisions must be made about treatments or interventions to sustain or prolong life. Health care "quality of life" assessments, therefore, focus on the physiological and mental conditions that limit or enhance the (incompetent) patient's life experiences for others to reach a judgment about whether the "burdens" of particular life-extending medical interventions are in that patient's "best interests" (i.e., are outweighed by the "benefits" of life-extension in these circumstances).

Quickening: In pregnancy, the moment at which the movement of the fetus in the uterus is first felt or perceived by the pregnant woman, usually occurring between eighteen and twenty-one weeks of pregnancy. Historically, the point of quickening has been applied in some theological and legal contexts (including the English common law) to identify that point at which the developing fetus is regarded as an individual human life.

Quinlan case: 1976 New Jersey Supreme Court case [*In re Quinlan,* 355 A.2D 647 (N.J. 1976)] that was the first major U.S. court decision allowing discontinuation of life-prolonging treatment for an incompetent individual. Karen Quinlan stopped breathing and lapsed into a coma in 1975 and was later diagnosed as being in a **persistent vegetative state.** Her father sought court permission to have her **ventilator** support withdrawn, allowing her to die. The Supreme Court of New Jersey found in favor of Mr. Quinlan, holding that Karen's individual right of privacy includes the right to accept or reject life-prolonging treatment. The court held further that life support may be removed if physicians and a "hospital ethics committee" agree that the patient will never return to a "cognitive, sapient state" and allowed Karen's guardian and family to determine whether she would choose to have the ventilator support withdrawn. After she was weaned from the ventilator, Karen continued to breathe spontaneously and survived for nine years.

❧ R ❧

Randomization: In medical **experimentation,** the process of determining by chance (rather than deliberate choice) the assignment of each subject to a particular treatment (or non-treatment) group within the research study. This is undertaken to minimize attitudinal or expectational bias among subjects or researchers and, in many therapeutic experimental trials, to ensure that each participant-subject has an equal chance of receiving that form of treatment that will be proven most effective.

Rationing: A process, policy, or method for the allocation or distribution of a needed resource when demand for that resource exceeds supply. (See also **allocation**)

"Reasonable person" standard: A legal standard with roots in the English common law tradition for assessing and evaluating the propriety of an individual's behavior on the basis of what a hypothetical ideal "reasonable person" would know or do, especially in cases involving allegations of negligence. In health care law, the reasonable person standard is applied in many U.S. states and jurisdictions in assessing the kind and amount of information (about potential risks, benefits, etc.) that must be disclosed to a patient for that individual to give genuine **informed consent** to recommended treatment (an "informed patient" standard) or for an individual to give genuine informed consent to be a subject of medical **experimentation** (a "reasonable subject" standard). As a standard for adequate disclosure of information in the informed consent

141

process, the reasonable person standard has competed (in the United States) with the "professional practice" standard, sometimes called the "reasonable doctor" standard, which would determine adequate disclosure of information on the basis of customary practices within the professional community. In contrast to the professional practice standard, the reasonable person standard evaluates the adequacy of information disclosed from the perspective of the patient's (or subject's) informational needs. Both standards involve significant ambiguity and lack of specificity because the point of reference is not the actual knowledge, abilities, or needs of any particular patient/subject or health professional but rather assumptions about what a "reasonable" person would need to know in the given patient's or subject's situation or what a "reasonable" professional ought to disclose in that particular situation. It is often pointed out, however, that the patient-focus of the reasonable person standard does encourage physicians and researchers to discuss proposed treatments or experiments with the patient/subject in a more thorough manner.

Recessive gene: A gene whose physical expression or trait (**phenotype**) is manifest only when the same **allele** for that gene is inherited from both parents (or, in the case of some genes on the X chromosome, only when the "normal" allele is not also present on another X chromosome—i.e., in a male, who has inherited one X and one Y chromosome). (See also **disorder, genetic**)

Recombinant DNA technology: A technique for creating new artificial **DNA** sequences resulting from the combination of two other DNA sequences (taken from different biological sources). These new DNA sequences can then be inserted into cells of organisms to become part of their **genome,** thus leading to the development of **genetically modified organisms.** Recombinant DNA technology has been used to produce genetically modified plants, vaccines, and peptide hormone medications such as insulin and **growth hormone.**

Relativism, ethical: This theory holds that all standards of moral rightness and wrongness are relative to the norms of one's culture or the society in which one is acting. In this view there are no objective or universal moral standards, so practices within a given society can be judged only against that society's standards.

Relativism, moral: The view that there exists no single standard for assessing the truth of any moral claim and thus that moral propositions cannot claim universal or absolute legitimacy but instead have meaning and truth only in relation to particular social, historical, cultural, or personal conventions. In contrast to *moral pluralism* (or value pluralism), which recognizes conflicting value-claims without holding that they are equally valid, moral relativism holds that opposing moral positions have no objective truth-value and no single standard of reference for judging between them.

Reproduction: The biological process by which new individual organisms are brought into being from existing organisms. The two main types of reproduction are sexual and asexual reproduction. In asexual reproduction, an organism creates another organism genetically identical or similar to itself without the contribution of any other organism. Sexual reproduction, on the other hand, is a process in which new organisms are produced from two parent organisms. Each parent organism contributes half of the genetic makeup of the offspring organism via **gametes** (e.g., egg and sperm cells) carrying **haploid** sets of chromosomes; they merge to form a **diploid** set of chromosomes in the cells of the offspring organism.

Reproductive cloning: Implanting a (cloned) organism into a woman's uterus with the goal of pregnancy and childbirth. The first reported successful reproductive cloning of a mammal via **SCNT** was a sheep, known to the world as "Dolly," born in 1997. (See **cloning**)

Required request: Term used for the requirement in various U.S. state and federal statutes that families of persons diagnosed as meeting the criteria of **brain death** be asked about their willingness to donate the deceased's organs or tissues for purposes of **transplantation.** The most broadly based application of "required request" legislation occurred with the federal Omnibus Budget Reconciliation Act of 1986, which states that any hospital receiving federal funding must give families of brain-dead persons the option of donating the deceased's organs. Prior to the enactment of required request statutes, public policy regarding cadaver organ retrieval in the United States had focused upon the right of individuals to elect (prospectively) donation of their own organs after death, as set forth in the **Uniform Anatomical Gift Act.** However, chronic shortages of cadaver organ supply (relative to demand) led to the addition of a focus upon family choice for/against donation in the "required request" approach.

Research protocol: See **protocol, research**

Restriction enzyme (or restriction endonuclease):   An enzyme that can cut through both strands of the double-helix DNA, yielding intact segments of DNA that may then be spliced together to form new and different DNA segments.

Restriction enzymes are critical to the technology of **genetic engineering.**

Retrovirus: A type of virus (of the viral family *Retroviridae*) containing strands of **RNA** within a protein shell. When a body cell is infected by a retrovirus, the viral RNA within the cell undergoes transcription (enabled by an enzyme, reverse transcriptase), which yields complementary strands of **DNA** that are in turn incorporated into the **genome** of the host cell so that the viral DNA is reproduced as part of that genome. The term "retrovirus" refers to the phenomenon of viral RNA being transcribed to produce DNA strands rather than complementary RNA strands. The **human immunodeficiency virus (HIV)** is an example of a retrovirus.

Rhythm method: A form of **natural family planning** in which prevention of conception and pregnancy is accomplished by periodic abstinence from sexual activity during those periods of a woman's menstrual cycle in which fertility is expected based upon the "rhythm" of her cycle of menstruation.

Ribonucleic acid (RNA):   A chemical (nucleic acid) similar in structure to **DNA,** found in the nucleus and cytoplasm of cells. RNA plays a vital role in the translation of the genetic code of the DNA nucleotide chain into structural proteins that give the cell (and the organism) its shape and functions. There are several different types of RNA molecules, including messenger RNA (mRNA), transfer RNA (tRNA), and ribosomal RNA (rRNA), each serving a different individual purpose.

Ribosome: A minute particle in the cytoplasm (cellular fluid) inside a cell (but outside its nucleus) containing protein and **RNA** and serving in the synthesis of proteins through a process called "translation" in which messenger RNA directs the sequence of amino acids in the growing polypeptide chains that form proteins.

Rights: Justifiable or supportable claims that one person or group can make against others. *Negative rights* are "liberties"— that is, claims against others not to restrain or interfere with one's own choices, actions, or interests. (The first ten amendments to the U.S. Constitution delineate a list of negative rights, for example.) *Positive rights* (or "entitlements"), conversely, are claims upon others for assistance in accomplishing one's chosen course of action or protecting one's interests. Generally, then, rights create (and depend upon) obligations on the part of others to respect those claims, either through noninterference or through positive assistance. Furthermore, rights may be distinguished as to the source of their justification: *Moral rights* are claims justified according to accepted moral norms (which specify the duties or obligations of others to respect those rights); *legal rights*, conversely, are claims justified according to the particular liberties and entitlements (and correlative obligations) specified in enacted laws or judicial interpretation of laws.

Right to die: A phrase, popular since the 1970s, denoting the freedom persons should have to reject life-prolonging treatments they do not desire. More recently, "right to die" has also referred to the claim by some to an entitlement to assistance in bringing about one's own death through the actions or assistance of others. The phrase became familiar with the 1976 New Jersey Supreme Court case regarding Karen Ann Quinlan, a young woman in a **persistent vegetative state (PVS)** whose parents claimed (successfully) that she would not choose, if able, to be kept alive in her present state, and that continued use of life support (specifically, a mechanical ventilator) would be against her will and a violation of her right to refuse unwanted medical treatment. In a later U.S. Supreme Court case (*Cruzan v. Director, Missouri Department of Health,* 110 S.Ct. 2841 [1990]) involving Nancy Cruzan, another young woman in PVS whose parents also sought removal of life-support (nutrition and hydration, in this case), the court's majority held that all citizens have a constitutional right to refuse life-prolonging treatment, extending even beyond the point at which they are no longer able to communicate their choices (provided there is sufficient evidence of those choices). However, in two 1997 cases (**Vacco v. Quill** and **Washington v. Glucksberg**) the Supreme Court held that the freedom to allow death by refusing life-prolonging treatment does not imply any positive entitlement to receive assistance in causing or hastening one's death via the positive actions of others (e.g., through physician-assisted **suicide** or active **euthanasia**). Nevertheless, some continue to argue for a moral right to such assistance, at least for terminally ill persons, based upon the moral principles of **beneficence** toward the dying and respect for the **autonomy** of that person and her wishes.

RNA: See **ribonucleic acid**

Roe v. Wade: Controversial U.S. Supreme Court case whose majority decision, issued in January 1973, required liberalization of most state **abortion** laws in effect at that time. The majority opinion, written by Justice Harry Blackmun, describes three legitimate "interests" which must be respected in formulating abortion statutes: a woman's right to privacy, including privacy with regard to reproductive decisions; the state's legitimate interest in preserving and protecting the health of pregnant women; and the state's legitimate interest in protecting "potential" (fetal) life. The opinion went on to claim that each of these interests becomes "compelling" at a particular stage of pregnancy. In the first trimester (roughly twelve weeks) of pregnancy, the states must assume that the most compelling interest at stake is the mother's right to privacy in reproductive decisions (including abortion) alone. The state's interest in protecting maternal health (along with her right to privacy) becomes compelling at the beginning of the second trimester of pregnancy, when abortion procedures become more complicated and risky to maternal health. And the state's interest in protecting potential life becomes compelling at the beginning of the third trimester of pregnancy, which (at that time) was considered also to coincide with the point of fetal **viability.** (However, the state's interest in protecting potential life could not outweigh the state's prior interest in protecting maternal health. Thus, the states could not prohibit abortion even in the third trimester of pregnancy in cases where the life or health of the mother would be jeopardized without the abortion procedure.) (*Roe v. Wade*, 410 U.S. 113 [1973].)

RU-486:   See **mifepristone**

Rule-utilitarianism: A theory of moral justification that holds that we ought always to act according to those rules of practice that will predictably yield the greatest overall good consequences (and least bad consequences) for all concerned if those rules are consistently followed. (See **utilitarianism**)

✺ S ✺

Schiavo case: A lengthy, much–publicized legal and ethical controversy regarding the withdrawal of life-prolonging treatment (specifically, artificially provided nutrition and hydration) from a Florida woman incapable of expressing her own wishes regarding treatment. Theresa Marie Schindler ("Terri") Schiavo, twenty–six years old, collapsed and lost consciousness in her home on February 26, 1990. She experienced cardiac and respiratory arrest resulting in significant brain damage from ischemia (lack of oxygenated blood supply). After two and a half months in a **coma,** she progressed into a sleep–wake cycle but did not exhibit any consistent or repeatable awareness of her environment or herself. Her condition was diagnosed by several consulting physicians as a **persistent vegetative state (PVS).** Unable to ingest food or liquids by mouth, she was fed initially via a **nasogastric tube,** then via a **PEG** tube. Her husband, Michael Schiavo, filed and won a malpractice lawsuit against Terri's obstetrician-gynecologist for failing to diagnose bulimia (which, it was charged, may have led to electrolyte imbalance and cardio-respiratory arrest in her case). After several years of extensive rehabilitation therapy programs and experimental treatments, Terri's condition had not changed and her husband filed a court petition (in 1998) requesting that her feeding tube be removed. Her parents strongly opposed his petition, arguing in part that Terri was a devout Roman Catholic and would consider refusal of nutrition/hydration to be a violation of Church teachings. After a trial in early 2000, the court determined that Terri, who had not created an **advance directive**

for health care, had made reliable oral statements indicating that she would want the feeding tube removed in her current circumstances. Her parents appealed this ruling; they also challenged Michael Schiavo's guardianship of Terri and later challenged her diagnosis of PVS and argued that new therapies could help restore her cognitive function. However, the initial court decision was upheld by several decisions of the Florida Second District Court of Appeal and the Supreme Court of Florida. (During this period Terri's feeding tube was removed once by court order, then replaced as part of the appeals process.) In early 2003 Terri's parents enlisted the aid of "pro-life" activists to publicize their daughter's situation and to lobby for other interventions that would keep Terri alive. After their judicial appeals were exhausted and Terri's feeding tube had been removed for the second time in October 2003, the Florida legislature passed "Terri's Law," which would permit the Florida governor to intervene by issuing a stay of feeding tube removal in cases like hers. Gov. Jeb Bush signed the bill and then ordered replacement of Terri's feeding tube. However, "Terri's Law" was found unconstitutional by Florida's 6th Circuit Court and by the Supreme Court of Florida in 2004, and the U.S. Supreme Court declined to review the case in early 2005. On March 18, 2005, Terri's feeding tube was removed for the third time. Three days later the U.S. Senate and House of Representatives passed via voice vote, and President George Bush immediately signed, a law allowing Terri's parents to take their case to the federal courts. Over the next nine days, however, their complaints and appeals were rejected by the federal courts, including the U.S. Supreme Court. Terri Schiavo died on March 31, 2005. An autopsy revealed extensive brain damage but could not determine the cause of her original collapse and ischemic brain injury. While the fundamental issues addressed by the courts in the early Schiavo petitions, hearings, and appeals were not unique or even unusual, the degree (and acrimony) of journalistic and public controversy in the case—coupled with the unprecedented legislative and executive involvements at both state and federal levels—was extraordinary. The case stimulated public responses from a remarkable array of sources. Perhaps the most famous (and most controversial) response came from Pope John Paul II, who in a March 2004 speech announced that the traditional Catholic distinction between **"extraordinary" and "ordinary" means of treatment** could not justify the withholding or withdrawing of artificial nutrition and hydration (as "extraordinary" means) from persons in persistent vegetative states. In his interpretation of the tradition and its modern application, the provision of nutrition and hydration, even by artificial means, must be considered a "natural" act and not a "medical" procedure. Furthermore, provision of nutrition and hydration must be considered "ordinary" insofar as it can accomplish the goals of providing nourishment and/or relieving suffering, even if it cannot bring about restoration of consciousness or other functions.

Schloendorff v. Society of the New York Hospital: A New York court case (105 N.E. 192 [N.Y. 1914]) that is often cited as the earliest expression of the legal doctrine of **informed consent** in the United States. The plaintiff in this case, Mary Schloendorff, claimed that she had consented only to an examination of her gangrenous arm and not the amputation of several fingers that followed that examination. While the court did not find the hospital liable, Justice Cardozo's opinion included the now-famous claim that every "human being of adult years and sound mind has a right to determine what shall be done with his own body."

SCNT (somatic cell nuclear transfer): See **cloning**

Self-determination, individual: The capacity, freedom, and **right** to choose and act in accordance with one's own values, beliefs, and commitments (at least within the limits of others' exercise of self-determination as well). The term is sometimes used as a synonym for **autonomy.**

Seroconversion: The change of an individual's **serostatus** from negative to positive—that is, the presence in the blood serum of detectable **antibodies** to a particular microorganism resulting from infection by that microorganism or from immunization using a killed, altered, or attenuated form of that microorganism.

Serostatus: The presence or absence in an individual's blood serum of **antibodies** that would signal the body's immune response to a particular **antigen** (often a virus, bacterium, or other infectious agent). So, for example, a person whose blood serum contains antibodies for the HIV virus would be seropositive (HIV+) for that antibody (and viral antigen); one whose blood serum has no trace of those antibodies would be seronegative for HIV (HIV−).

Sex-linked disorder: See **disorder, genetic**

Sex preselection: A form of **sex selection** undertaken prior to conception or prior to the establishment of pregnancy, using sperm separation techniques or genetic diagnostic techniques along with **assisted reproductive technology.** One form of sex preselection strategy involves separating sperm bearing the Y-chromosome from sperm bearing the (heavier) X-chromosome through a technique called flow cytometric separation; then a concentrated sample of the preferred sperm group is used, via artificial insemination, to bring about fertilization, pregnancy, and birth of a child of the preferred sex.

Alternatively, when fertilization has been accomplished via **in vitro fertilization, preimplantation genetic diagnosis** may be employed to determine the sex (and other genetic character-istics) of the very early embryo (**morula**); then an embryo of the desired sex may be selected for transfer to the mother's uterus for implantation, pregnancy, and birth.

Sex selection: The use of genetic diagnostic techniques and **assisted reproductive technology** (whether preconcep-tion, preimplantation, or prenatal) for purposes of ensuring the probability or actuality of delivering a child of the sex selected by the parents (or preventing the implantation or birth of a child not of the desired sex).

Sexual reproduction: See **reproduction**

Siamese twins: archaic term for **conjoined twins**. (See **twins**)

Sickle cell disease (or sickle cell anemia or hemoglobin ss disease):   A genetic disease in which the body produces abnormal crescent or sickle-shaped red blood cells that can clump together and restrict blood flow in organs and tissues (causing pain and lack of tissue oxygenation) and that dete-riorate more quickly than normal red blood cells (causing **anemia**). Sickle cell disease is a homozygous recessive auto-somal disorder, meaning that the gene **allele** for the disease must be inherited from both parents for the disease to be manifest in the offspring. Offspring who are heterozygous for the sickle cell gene (i.e., inherited the disease gene allele from one parent and the "normal" gene allele from the other) are said to have sickle cell trait, which usually involves no disease symptoms (except in rare cases). The sickle cell gene is most commonly found in populations (and descendant popula-tions) from Africa, from areas surrounding the Mediterranean

Sea, and from some Spanish-speaking areas in South America, Central America, and the Caribbean. **Genetic screening** for the sickle cell gene is required for newborn infants in more than forty U.S. states. In modern U.S. history, many mandatory state and federal mass sickle cell screening programs (for young children, persons seeking marriage licenses, and inmates in prisons and mental institutions, for example) have been criticized (and often repealed) as racially or ethnically discriminatory policies.

Single-gene disorder: Disorders due to a "mistake" at single gene location on a given **chromosome.** (See **disorder, genetic**)

Single-payer system: A system of health care financing in which all health care costs are paid for by a single (governmental) agency, usually funded through taxation. The practices of health care providers and the operation of institutions may remain private, but all reimbursement for care provided comes from a single source. In the Canadian single-payer model, for instance, physicians are reimbursed according to a rate scale negotiated yearly with Provincial officials; hospitals may be privately managed but are financed via global budgets from the single funding source. (See also **socialized medicine**)

Situationalism: Term used to describe the stance taken by those advocating and practicing **situation ethics.**

Situation ethics: A theory or method of moral reasoning and justification that gives decisive weight to the circumstances or "situation" in judging whether a particular action is right or wrong. Its most famous proponent, Joseph Fletcher, argued in his *Situation Ethics* (1966) that situation ethics is a "third approach" to moral reasoning, along with "legalism" (rigid adherence to strict moral rules with no regard to the possible negative consequences of doing so) and "antinomianism" (a complete rejection of all moral principles, rules, guidelines, etc.). In Fletcher's view, one and only one moral principle is final and absolute—*agape*, the norm of neighbor-love heralded in Christianity. Furthermore, Fletcher's agape amounts to loving one's neighbors by always acting to produce the "greatest good for the greatest number" of neighbors (a definition that brings Fletcher's approach close to that form of **consequentialism** known as **act-utilitarianism**). Thus, for Fletcher, choosing the morally right course of action is a matter of applying reason to a simple assessment of "love plus the situation." It follows, too, that any particular act could be morally justifiable (indeed, obligatory) given the circumstances of the particular situation in which it is performed.

Slippery-slope argument: Also called a **wedge argument,** a claim that the moral acceptance of some types of (previously impermissible) actions will lead to other acts or practices that cannot be similarly justified and should not be accepted. One version of the slippery-slope argument focuses on logical consistency in ethical arguments and suggests that if we accept an act in circumstance A but cannot provide good moral reasons why circumstance A is relevantly dissimilar to circumstance B, then we must accept the same act or practice in circumstance B, even if that act in that circumstance strikes us as morally wrong. (For example, some claim that moral or legal acceptance of voluntary active euthanasia in certain specific circumstances, such as extreme suffering in terminal illness, may lead to its application in other circumstances that do not now strike us as justifiable but may nevertheless be claimed to be relevantly similar circumstances.) The other form of wedge or slippery-slope argument focuses on the psychological or sociological context in which the act or practice in question would be accepted and employed and questions whether other social or cultural attitudes or forces might not lead to expansion of that act or practice in unacceptable ways. For example, using the same scenario cited above, some might argue that social acceptance of voluntary active euthanasia, even in very limited circumstances, may lead to a much more permissive attitude toward and acceptance of active euthanasia due to social forces such as racism, bias toward the aged and those with defects requiring expensive care, or simply the sense of ease and familiarity that grows with repetition of the practice over time. Put in other words, if our moral obligation to respect and protect innocent human life has been expressed thus far through rules that would, among other things, prohibit active euthanasia, then we may be risking erosion of our ultimate sense of respect for human life by making exceptions to those rules against taking life—especially as those presumably justifiable exceptions begin to multiply in number.

Socialized medicine: A term used (often pejoratively) to describe systems of public, governmental organization, administration, financing, or delivery of health care services. In any genuinely "socialized" system of health care, providers would be employed by government, hospitals and institutions would be owned and operated by government, and financing would be provided by government through tax revenues. Yet, some critics expand the category of socialized health care systems to include single-payer national health insurance schemes (like the Canadian system), which are more accurately "socialized health insurance" systems.

Somatic cell: A cell from any part of the body (soma) that is not a **germ cell** (or **gamete**)—that is, all body cells except sperm and ova.

Somatic cell gene therapy: See **gene therapy**

Somatic cell nuclear transfer (SCNT): A procedure in which the nucleus from a somatic (nonreproductive) cell of an individual is transferred into an unfertilized ovum (egg cell) whose nucleus (containing the maternal chromosomes) has been removed; the ovum is then stimulated to begin dividing, leading to the development of a new organism with the same chromosomal complement (genome) as the individual from whom the somatic cell nucleus was taken. (See also **cloning**)

Somatropin (or somatotrophin): A polypeptide hormone produced in the anterior pituitary gland that stimulates cell reproduction and body growth. (See **growth hormone**)

Speciesism: A term coined by Richard D. Ryder in 1973 to connote discriminatory and prejudicial attitudes toward, and treatment of, individuals based upon the (allegedly irrelevant) criterion of their membership in particular species. The charge of speciesism is used most often by animal rights advocates as a criticism of those who ascribe lesser moral status, value, and rights to nonhuman animals, comparing this form of interspecies discrimination to racism and sexism among individuals within the human species. (See, e.g., Peter Singer, *Animal Liberation,* 2nd ed. [New York: New York Review of Books/Random House, 1990].)

Sperm bank: See **germplasm bank**

Sperm donation: See **gamete donation**

Spermatozoon: A male reproductive cell (sperm).

Spina bifida: A **neural tube defect** in which a malformation of the vertebrae (backbones) allows for protrusion and exposure of the spinal cord. This condition is caused by a failure of the neural tube (the embryonic structure that forms the brain and spinal cord) to fully close during embryonic development. Symptoms of spina bifida include incontinence of bladder and bowel, learning disabilities, and limited mobility.

Spontaneous abortion: Miscarriage; an unplanned, nondeliberate, noninduced evacuation of a fetus from a pregnant woman's uterus.

Stakeholders: Term now common in business ethics coined by the Stanford Research Institute in the 1960s to denote the various persons and groups that provide critical support to a business organization. Applied to health care organizations, the term would refer to all those who support or can affect or be affected by the organization's achievement of its purposes or objectives. These would include not only patients, on the one hand, and owners or administrators, on the other, but also clinical professionals, support staff and other employees, business partners and contractors, and the community within which the organization seeks to function. (See, e.g., W. Evan and R. Freeman, "A Stakeholder Theory of the Modern Corporation: Kantian Capitalism," in T. Beauchamp and N. Bowie, eds., *Ethical Theory and Business,* 3rd ed. [Englewood Cliffs, N.J.: Prentice Hall, 1988], pp. 97–106.)

State medicine: A term, roughly synonymous with **socialized medicine,** referring to health care systems that are organized and operated through government agencies and with public financing. Some have also used the term, disparagingly, in reference to proposals for single-payer national health insurance schemes, governmental regulation of pharmaceutical marketing/manufacturing, and other broad regulatory policies restricting free-market practices in health care economics.

Stem cells: Specialized cells within the body that are distinct from other cells in two important ways: They are not yet specialized or differentiated (that is, destined to be only one kind of cell with one kind of function) and can reproduce themselves almost indefinitely through cell division; and, second, they can be induced under certain conditions to differentiate into particular types or lines of cells (e.g., into pancreatic cells that will secrete insulin). Thus, stem cells can function to repair or replace cells and tissues that are lost or malfunctioning due to disease, injury, or abnormal development. In the **embryonic development** of human beings, the early clump of four to eight cells exhibits **totipotency** (that is, any one of these cells could be separated and induced to form a complete embryo and placenta, amniotic sac, etc.). By three to five days after conception, the spherical **blastocyst** contains **embryonic stem cells** in its hollow center; these cells are **pluripotent** (i.e., capable of forming any kind of tissue within the body of the embryo itself but not the external placenta or amniotic sac). Stem cells also exist in the bodies of persons after birth, in the bone marrow, brain, and muscle, for example. The umbilical cord blood of newborns is especially rich in stem cells. These latter types of stem cells, **adult stem cells,** are **multipotent** (that is, they are capable of developing into several lines of cells and tissues in body). Recent experiments also raise the possibility of "de-differentiating" normal adult cells (that is, inducing them to revert to a more stem-cell-like multipotent or pluripotent state). The range of possible therapeutic uses of stem cells is enormous. And applications of adult stem cell therapies (bone marrow transplantation, for example) seem to raise no ethical concerns so long as their retrieval causes no harm to their (consenting) donors. However, there is much controversy surrounding the harvesting of embryonic stem cells (which many scientists regard as more therapeutically promising because of their pluripotency). For retrieval of these cells requires the destruction of embryonic blastocysts that have been created through **in vitro fertilization** and are "left over" from reproductive attempts or were created specifically for stem cell harvesting. And for those who believe that human life and human personhood begin at conception, destruction of early embryos for this or any other purpose is murder and cannot be morally justified, regardless of its therapeutic value to others.

Sterilization: In human/animal biology, the process of rendering an individual unable to procreate due to disease, radiation, or surgical or chemical intervention. Surgical sterilization may be accomplished via **hysterectomy** (removal of the uterus), **oophorectomy** (removal of the ovaries), or **orchiectomy** (castration, removal of the testes). **Vasectomy** (tying off the male vasa deferentia) and **tubal ligation** (tying off the female fallopian tubes) are forms of reversible surgical sterilization or, more accurately, reversible "permanent contraception."

Substituted judgment: A legal (and moral) standard for decision making regarding consent for the treatment or research participation of a person who is not competent to give his own consent (but has been competent in the past). According to this standard, **surrogate consent** on behalf of the presently incompetent individual should be based upon the surrogate having sufficient knowledge of the beliefs, values, fears, and aspirations of that individual to confidently predict what he would choose if he were currently competent and able to choose. In other words, the surrogate should be able to answer the question, "What would this patient want in this situation?"

Suicide: The death of an individual resulting from that person's deliberate act or omission chosen with the intent of ending her life. Thus, the individual who commits suicide must not only knowingly choose a course of action or omission likely to lead to her death but must also intend death as a consequence of that choice. In **assisted suicide** the individual who has chosen to die is assisted by another person who, for example, may provide advice or information about how best to accomplish self-killing or may provide the means necessary to do so. Social and legal acceptance of **physician-assisted suicide (PAS)** has been a subject of great debate in the United States since the early 1990s. While many states have held public referenda regarding the legalization of PAS, only Oregon and Washington have legalized it, with many restrictions and only in cases of terminal illness.

Supererogatory: Ancient term meaning "above and beyond [one's] moral obligation." (See **beneficence**)

Superovulation: Development and release of multiple ova (eggs) at the same time by the ovaries. Superovulation therapy, frequently employed in the treatment of female infertility, utilizes hormones and other drugs to induce superovulation.

Surrogate consent: A replacement or substitution for an individual's own **informed consent** to treatment or research participation, given by another person acting as surrogate for that individual because he is incompetent or otherwise incapable of consent. Several standards have been asserted in both legal and moral contexts for the content of decision making in surrogate consent. First, if the now–incompetent individual has made known previously (while competent) his own autonomous wishes regarding the kind of consent at stake, then those expressions should guide the surrogate's current consent or nonconsent. Second, when the previously competent individual has made known no explicit preferences that would guide the consent decision but has established clear patterns of life preferences, values, goals, and objectives, then the surrogate's task would be to use that life history to choose as the now–incompetent person would have chosen—a standard referred to as **substituted judgment.** In the case of the incompetent individual who was never competent or whose previous life patterns and choices are largely unknown, the remaining standard for surrogate consent decisions is the **best interests standard,** reflecting an objective assessment of the kind of consent a reasonable person would probably give for himself in these circumstances (or perhaps also building upon subjective valuations expressed by the incompetent individual in the past that may seem relevant in the present). Many legal jurisdictions have also enacted statutes specifying who should be empowered to give surrogate consent on behalf of an incompetent person who has not previously identified her own preferred surrogate.

Surrogate gestation: The implantation in a woman's uterus of an embryo not genetically related to her so that she undergoes pregnancy and delivers the infant on behalf of other, genetic or adoptive, parents.

Surrogate mother: A woman who enters into a contract in which she agrees to undergo pregnancy on behalf of another woman (who is unable or unwilling to conceive or gestate). Her pregnancy may occur via natural or artificial insemination (in which case she is also the donor of the egg, and thus

the genetic as well as gestational mother of the infant conceived) or via in vitro fertilization with embryo transfer (in
cases where the egg is donated by the contracting/adoptive
mother or by a third party egg donor; see **assisted reproductive
technology**). The sperm donor is usually the husband or partner
of the contracting/adoptive mother. The surrogate mother
contracts to surrender parental rights to the contracting/
adoptive parents after birth although some state laws require
a waiting period during which she may decide to void the
contract and claim maternal rights to the newborn.

Syndrome: In medicine and psychology, a set of symptoms, signs, or manifestations that occur frequently together
so that the presence of one often signals the presence of the
others. A syndrome may or may not be identified as being
caused by a specific disease, disorder, or condition.

$\backsim\!\!T\!\!\backsim$

Tarasoff case: 1976 California Supreme Court case (*Tarasoff v. Regents of the University of California,* California Supreme Court, 17 California Reports, 3d series, 425, decided July 1, 1976) in which the majority opinion recognized a legal **duty to warn** that may override a mental health therapist's traditional duty to maintain **confidentiality** of "privileged" patient information in cases where the patient poses a credible, probable risk of harm to an identifiable third party. In this case, a patient had confided to his treating psychologist that he intended to kill his fiancée when she returned from a trip to another country. The psychologist initially requested that university police detain the patient but then decided not to seek the patient's commitment for observation in a mental hospital because that request would entail sharing information revealed confidentially during therapy. The patient's fiancée, unaware of any threat to her well-being, returned to her home and shortly thereafter was killed by the patient. In the California Supreme Court's majority opinion, public interest in the protection of innocent, unsuspecting victims from violent assault must outweigh the public importance of protecting patient confidentiality. Thus, therapists who are made aware of and are convinced of the seriousness of a patient's intent to harm an identifiable other party have a duty to ensure that that other party is warned of the nature of the threat. While the Tarasoff case applied only to California jurisdictions, all fifty U.S. states have adopted, via legal precedents or statute law, some version of the duty to warn established in *Tarasoff v. Regents of the University of California.*

Tay-Sachs disease: A rare genetic disease (a recessive **autosomal disorder**) that is fatal in its most common, infantile type. It is caused by mutations on a gene on chromosome 15, and is characterized by a buildup of the GM2 ganglioside (a fatty acid derivative) in the nerve cells of the brain. It is most common among Ashkenazi Jewish populations from Eastern Europe although it has been identified in other populations as well. Most commonly, infants born with Tay-Sachs disease will appear to develop normally for about six months but then experience deterioration of mental and physical abilities leading to blindness, deafness, inability to swallow, muscle atrophy and paralysis, and death by age four or five years. Tay-Sachs was one of the first genetic diseases for which widespread **genetic screening** was undertaken, using an inexpensive enzyme assay test. Testing and genetic counseling regarding Tay-Sachs disease has been widespread among Ashkenazi Jews (and in the State of Israel), leading to virtual elimination of instances of the disease in that population.

Teleology: Traditionally, the philosophical study of the purposes, ends, or directive principles in nature or in human actions or inventions (from the Greek *telos*, meaning "end" or "purpose"). As a theory of moral justification, a teleology will hold that every human action must be judged right or wrong according to its promotion of proper human ends or purposes, or (in consequentialist forms of teleology) according to the goodness or badness of its predicted consequences. So, for example, Roman Catholic **natural law** theory holds that certain natural purposes, tendencies, or inclinations (*inclinationes naturales*) are imprinted upon all of nature and are readily discernible through human rationality. These basic tendencies thus constitute our basic human values, and morally right actions will be those that promote (or at least do not deny) these values. Conversely, **consequentialism** constitutes another form of moral teleology in which the right action is always the action that will (predictably) result in the greatest overall balance of "good" consequences over "evil" consequences for the greatest number of persons affected. (This requires, of course, some form of value-theory by which the "goodness" or "badness" of consequences might be assessed in the first place.)

Teratogen: A chemical or other agent or influence that causes physical defects in the developing embryo or fetus.

Teratoma: A type of tumor arising from a sperm or egg cell that may grow to contain several types of tissues and even elements of bone, muscle, or hair. Teratomas are most often found in the ovaries, testes, or in the tailbone area of children, and may be **benign** or **malignant.**

Tetraploidy: Having four **chromosomes** of a particular type, in contrast to the normal human condition of two chromosomes of each type (diploid) in body cells and one chromosome of each type (haploid) in sperm and ova cells. (See also **aneuploidy**)

Theocentric, theocentrism: A theological perspective focused on what may be discerned about the will and purposes of divine powers, as opposed to an *anthropocentric* perspective focused upon the perceived welfare and well-being of human beings. (See, e.g., James M. Gustafson, *Ethics from a Theocentric Perspective,* vols. I and II [Chicago: University of Chicago Press, 1981, 1984].)

Therapeutic abortion: In general terms, an induced abortion procured to preserve the life or health of the pregnant woman, to prevent the birth of an infant with serious genetic or other congenital abnormalities, or to selectively reduce the number of fetuses (via *multifetal pregnancy reduction*) in cases where the number of fetuses threatens the prospects for individual fetal viability or survivability. Therapeutic abortion is often contrasted with elective abortion. (See **abortion**)

Therapeutic cloning: Cloning undertaken to produce early embryos whose **stem cells** can be harvested for medical research and therapeutic purposes. (See **cloning**)

Therapeutic privilege (or therapeutic exception): A controversial legal exception to the normal requirements of **informed consent** in which a physician may be justified in withholding information from a patient regarding his diagnosis, prognosis, or treatment on the grounds that the patient is not emotionally or psychologically stable enough to handle the information, and thus that disclosure may pose a serious risk of harm to the patient.

Therapeutic research: Medical experimentation generally involving subjects who have some pathology or illness for which treatment is the issue under investigation. Therapeutic research has the twin aim of generating useful medical knowledge while also (hopefully) benefiting the patient-subjects by identifying a superior form of treatment for their condition. (See **experimentation, medical**)

Third-party consent: A term for **proxy** or **surrogate consent.**

Totality, principle of: Moral principle frequently invoked in Roman Catholic moral theology that states that the good of a part may be sacrificed to preserve the good of the whole. Applied to the human body, for example, Thomas Aquinas invoked this principle in his *Summa Theologiae* to justify the bodily "mutilation" of amputating a diseased limb for the sake of preserving the life of the body. The principle has been applied in Catholic justifications of (nonvital) organ donations from living donors through an interpretation of totality and "integrity" that holds that the "functional integrity" of the body may be maintained even if its "anatomical integrity" is damaged via removal of an organ. This reality, coupled with the charitable intentions of the donor, serves the spiritual and physical "totality" of that person. (See, e.g., Benedict M. Ashley, Jean deBlois, and Kevin D. O'Rourke, *Health Care Ethics*, 5th ed. [Washington, D.C.: Georgetown University Press, 2006].) Some interpretations of "totality" have been controversial, however, when the "whole" at stake has been defined to mean a social or community group rather than a single bodily entity.

Total parenteral nutrition (TPN):   A procedure for delivering all the body's nutritional requirements through a catheter inserted into a major vein (e.g., a **PICC** line) for persons who cannot swallow, digest, or absorb food taken orally. Another term often used as a synonym for TPN is **hyperalimentation.**

Totipotency: In biology, the ability of a single cell to divide and give rise to all the different cell types of a particular organism. (See **stem cells**)

TPN: See **total parenteral nutrition**

Transgenic animal: An animal that has had a foreign **gene** deliberately inserted into its **genome.** The foreign genetic material is constructed using **recombinant DNA technology,** then transferred into the animal (now a **genetically modified organism**), leading to the expression of new or modified traits in that animal.

Transplantation, organ and tissue: The removal of organs or other bodily tissues (e.g., bone marrow, corneas) from one individual for implantation into the body of another individual, or into another part of the donor individual's body. A transplant from one part of a person's body into another part of her body is called an autograft. A transplant of an organ or tissue between the bodies of two members of the same species is an **allograft,** whereas a transplant between members of different species is a xenograft or heterograft. The first successful human solid organ allograft (a kidney) in the United States occurred in Boston in 1954. While some graft procedures (surgeries for the implantation of organs taken from another body) can be complex, the most difficult aspect of transplantation technology is usually the "rejection phenomenon"—that is, the recipient's immune system's attack upon the implanted organ or tissue, which it recognizes as "foreign" protein. Indeed, the earliest successful kidney transplants were undertaken with identical twins as organ donor and organ recipient so that the implanted tissue would be recognized as genetically nonforeign by the recipient's immune system. Over time advances in **immunosuppression** therapies, especially with the availability of **cyclosporine** in the early 1980s, have allowed successful transplants between donors and recipients who are much more genetically dissimilar. While the number and range of types of technically feasible and medically indicated transplants has ballooned over the past few decades, the number of organs available for transplantation has not. Since the late 1960s, public policy in the United States has encouraged individual decisions to donate one's organs or tissues for transplantation after one's death through the **Uniform Anatomical Gift Act.** In the mid–1980s, in an attempt to increase the number of cadaver organs for transplant by focusing upon the deceased's family as the source of consent for organ retrieval, state legislatures and the federal government passed so-called **required request** statutes. More recently, some institutions have enacted policies allowing for **donation after cardiac death (DCD),** in which a dying individual who does not meet the usual organ-donor requirement of whole **brain death** is allowed to die under circumstances in which her organs may be removed immediately (with family consent). Also, while it was once possible to remove only a kidney, blood, or bone marrow from a living person for transplant purposes without grievous harm to the donor, it is now possible for a living individual to donate a lobe of a lung or liver, a part of a pancreas, and so on. This has increased the number of possible graft procedures and recipient survival rates. (In several recent years the number of living organ/tissue donors has surpassed the number of cadaver donors in the United States.) At the same time, however, it has led some to question the true "voluntariness" of consents from many living donors faced with family members or close friends in need of transplantable organs/tissues.

Transsexualism: Generally, a condition in which an individual self-identifies as the gender other than the gender assigned to that individual at birth.

Triage: From the French *trier*, to "sort" or "pick," the sorting or allocation of treatment of patients to maximize potential effectiveness of available health care resources in terms of positive health or survival outcomes among those patients. In wartime medical aid situations, community disasters, or overcrowded emergency departments or intensive care units, triage decisions usually give priority for immediate treatment (or bed access) to those seriously sick or injured but able to recover. The next group treated would be those with less serious injuries or illnesses whose treatment might safely be delayed, then those with minor injuries or illnesses (the "walking wounded"), and finally those most severely ill or injured persons for whom no treatment will likely be useful. Triage exhibits a form of **microallocation** or **rationing,** an allotment of a scarce resource among persons, focused upon the **utilitarian** aim of producing the most successful health outcomes for the greatest number of persons using the available resources most efficiently. Many critics of utilitarianism point out, however, that one danger in schemes of triage is that judgments of "medical utility" (potential medical usefulness for an individual) might begin to include judgments of "social utility" (the individual's perceived usefulness to the community and thus the community's interest in treating her preferentially).

Triploidy: See **aneuploidy**

Twins: In animal biology, a form of multiple birth in which the mother delivers two offspring from the same pregnancy. The most common type of twins, "fraternal" or **dizygotic twins,** result when two different fertilized eggs implant into the uterine wall at the same time. They have an extremely small chance of having the same genetic profile, and may look no more similar than other nontwin siblings. "Identical" or **monozygotic twins,** conversely, result when the **zygote** formed from the fertilization of a single egg by a single sperm splits, yielding two separate embryos with the same **genome.** If the zygote splits very early, within two days after fertilization in the human, the resulting twins will have separate placentas and amniotic sacs; if the split occurs later, then they will share a placenta but have separate amniotic sacs. In a very rare occurrence, "half-identical" monozygotic twins may result when a zygote splits after the fertilization of a single egg with two different sperm. **Conjoined twins** (or Siamese twins) are monozygotic twins whose bodies are joined together at birth. **Cloning** produces the equivalent of a time-delayed identical twin of the individual whose somatic cell nucleus is used in the cloning process.

ᔐ U ᔐ

UAGA: See **Uniform Anatomical Gift Act**

Ultrasonography, medical: Diagnostic technique using ultrasound (cyclic sound pressure with a frequency too high for human hearing) imaging techniques to visualize organs, muscles, and other internal structures in the body. A very common use of ultrasonography is to provide three-dimensional images of the fetus in pregnancy.

Uniform Anatomical Gift Act (UAGA): A collection of state statutes governing the donation of human organs for **transplantation.** The UAGA is an example of a "uniform act" or "model code"—that is, an attempt to harmonize state laws regarding a particular issue throughout the United States. The UAGA governs the process of individual decisions to make gifts of one's organs (after death) for purposes of transplantation or medical research; the identities of those persons who might make such gifts on behalf of a deceased person when no prior decision has been made by the deceased; limits of liability for health care providers who act on good faith representation that organ donation was the wish of the deceased; and so on. U.S. citizens are probably most familiar with the part of the UAGA that created a process for choosing to become an organ donor by completing a short form on a driver's license or state identity card.

Uniform Determination of Death Act (UDDA):   A "uniform act" (to harmonize or coordinate individual state laws) approved in 1980 by the (U.S.) National Conference of Commissioners on State Laws in cooperation with the American Bar Association, American Medical Association, and the President's Commission on Medical Ethics. Its aim is to "provide a comprehensive and medically sound basis for determining death in all situations." The UDDA has been adopted by most U.S. states. (See **brain death**)

Universalizability: A concept popularized by eighteenth-century German philosopher Immanuel Kant regarding the consistent applicability of norms (or "maxims") of moral conduct. As part of his first formulation of what he called the "categorical imperative" (in his *Groundwork of the Metaphysic of Morals*) Kant claimed that one should always act in such a way that she could will that the maxim from which she is acting should become a universal law for all to follow. More recent (and more simplified) versions of the criterion of universalizability in moral judgment focus on its similar-choices-in-similar-circumstances aspect. They assert, for example, that if a person judges action *x* to be morally right (or obligatory, or virtuous, etc.) in circumstance *y*, then she is committed to the premise that action *x* would also be right (or obligatory, or virtuous) in any other circumstance relevantly similar to circumstance *y* (i.e., any other circumstance that is not different from *y* in any morally relevant way).

Universal precautions: Practices and procedures employed by health care practitioners to prevent the spread of infectious diseases through consistent use of "barrier" protections (e.g., gloves, masks, goggles, gowns, shoe covers) in patient-care settings and contexts. With the identification in 1983 of the **human immunodeficiency virus (HIV)** as the cause of **AIDS,** and with the discovery that the virus is present in many body fluids of infected persons, new approaches were sought to minimize the spread of the virus via contact with those fluids by uninfected persons. Health care organizations in the United States and elsewhere began to recommend, and then require, policies of "universal precautions" mandating barrier protections to minimize contact between each patient's body fluids and care givers' (and others') skin or mucous membranes. These precautions were called "universal" because they were not to be followed only in cases where infection was known or suspected but in every situation of contact with the body fluids of another. In other words, health care workers were to interact with every patient as if he were known to be infected. Universal precautions policies have been credited with reducing the rate of transmission not only of HIV but also of hepatitis B and other blood-borne pathogens in health care settings.

Utilitarianism: A family of theories of moral justification that are generally regarded as forms of **teleology** and, more specifically, **consequentialism.** Simply put, utilitarian ethical theories always regard one principle or norm of morality as ultimate and final—the principle of utility. While "utility" has had a variety of definitions, most agree on the general assertion that one should always seek to produce the greatest possible balance of value (or "good") over disvalue (or "evil") for all involved. But utilitarian theories can differ on a number of points. For one, how do we define the "good" we are to maximize and the "evil" we are to avoid or minimize? Nineteenth-century British philosophers Jeremy Bentham and John Stuart Mill, regarded as the founders of utilitarianism, are often called *hedonistic* utilitarians in that they

conceived of utility as the maximization of happiness or pleasure. Indeed, Bentham frequently referred to the principle
of utility as the "pleasure principle." Other, later utilitarians,
however, insisted that basic goods or values are essentially
multiple and cannot be reduced simply to forms of happiness
or pleasure. Such theorists, such as philosopher G. E. Moore,
are thus regarded as *pluralistic* utilitarians. Yet other utilitarians hold that genuine value or good is subjectively perceived,
and thus one person's good may not be good for another but
must instead be defined in each circumstance according to
individual preference. These theorists are often referred to as
preferential utilitarians. Another major focus of differentiation
among utilitarian theories has to do with the question of how,
ultimately, utility is best maximized. Act-utilitarians argue that
we should always, in each particular situation of choice, actu-
alize utility by calculating the overall [probable] outcomes or
consequences of every course of action available to us and
then choose the one action that will predictably yield the
greatest net good for all involved (or, in crude terms, produce
"the greatest good for the greatest number"). **Act-utilitarianism**
is, then, frequently referred to as a form of **situation ethics**
because any identification of the "right" thing to do is fully
dependent upon an analysis of each unique situation or circumstance in which a choice must be made. **Rule-utilitarians,**
on the other hand, argue that individualized, situation-
restricted calculations of good and evil outcomes may not be
the best way to maximize utility overall. They recognize, for
example, a real value in social respect for rules of practice, and
the consistency and predictability of human actions following from that respect for rules. Thus they hold that we ought
always to act in accordance with the rule of practice that, if
generally followed, would yield the greatest overall balance
of good over evil for everyone involved. In this view, then,

social experience and reflection can illuminate for us those general rules (and context-dependent exceptions to those rules as well) that will probably yield the greatest overall utility if they are generally followed by all. Utility is best served, then, when we consistently follow those rules that have been shown to be utility-maximizing rules of practice.

ᔑ V ᔑ

Vacco v. Quill: 1997 U.S. Supreme Court case (521 U.S. 793 [1997]) regarding the question of an individual's right to seek and receive assistance in **suicide.** New York State law prohibits assisted suicide but permits patients' refusal of life-prolonging treatment. Physician–petitioners argued that this differentiation among death–resulting choices manifested a violation of the equal protection clause of the Fourteenth Amendment of the Constitution—that terminally ill persons dependent upon life-support devices are free to die via rejection of those treatments, whereas terminally ill persons who are not dependent upon such devices do not have the freedom to seek assistance in escaping their painful or oppressive conditions. The Supreme Court majority held that there is a clear and important distinction between *allowing* death from an underlying (untreated) condition and *intending* and *causing* death via assistance in suicide, and thus that treating the two situations differently in New York law does not violate the U.S. Constitution. (See also **Washington v. Glucksberg,** another case addressing assisted suicide rights and decided by the Supreme Court on the same day.)

Vector: A carrier that transfers an infectious agent from one organism to another. Also, a *viral* vector, consisting of a virus that has been altered to carry human DNA, is used to insert new DNA sequences (genes) into target cells in **gene therapy.**

Vegetative state: See **persistent vegetative state**

Ventilator, medical (or mechanical):   An automated machine used to deliver breathable air to and from the lungs of an individual who is unable to breathe or whose breathing capacity is not sufficient to maintain adequate oxygen supply to the body. Synonyms include "respirator" and "mechanical respirator."

Viability: In the terminology of biology, the state or quality of being able to maintain an independent existence (for an organism) and to live after birth.

Virology: The study of **viruses** and viral infections.

Virtue ethics: A theory of morality whose primary moral focus is upon character and moral virtues and excellences (arête in Greek). It is an ethics of being rather than an ethics of doing. That is, the central moral question for aretaic or virtue ethics is not "What should I do?" or "How should I judge that action?" but rather "What sort of person should I become, and what sorts of virtues should I manifest in living my life?" Aristotle referred to virtue as one's capacity to do well something that perfects his nature. (See, e.g., his *Nicomachean Ethics* [trans. Martin Ostwald, New York: Bobbs-Merrill, 1962]). A more modern definition of a moral virtue would be a trait, habit, or disposition that is morally valued—i.e., that leads one to live and act in a morally right or praiseworthy manner. In the Western Hippocratic tradition of medicine, certain virtues of the "good physician" have been emphasized repeatedly. These have included benevolence and nonmalevolence, fairness, respect for privacy and confidentiality, truthfulness, compassion, trustworthiness, faithfulness, prudence, and integrity. (See, e.g., Edmund G. Pellegrino,

"The Virtuous Physician and the Ethics of Medicine," in Earl Shelp, ed., *Virtue and Medicine* [Dordrecht: D. Reidel, 1985], and "Toward a Virtue-Based Normative Ethics for the Health Professions," *Kennedy Institute of Ethics Journal* 5 [1995]: 253–77; also Tom L. Beauchamp and James F. Childress, *Principles of Biomedical Ethics,* 6th ed. [New York: Oxford University Press, 2009], especially chapter 2.)

Virus: A tiny (submicroscopic) protein-based entity that can infect other more complex living cells and organisms. Structurally, the virus particle (or virion) contains nucleic acid, either **DNA** or **RNA,** surrounded by a protein shell (capsid). While viruses are like other living organisms in containing nucleic acids, they are unlike living organisms, even one-celled organisms, in their inability to divide, reproduce, or metabolize on their own, or to respond to changes in their environment. They can replicate only by infecting a host cell, whose own metabolic and replicative machinery produces multiple copies of the viral DNA or RNA.

Vitalism: As commonly employed in the literature of bioethics, a term referring to the belief that the preservation and extension of human biological life (generally regardless of the conditions of that life) is a basic, fundamental, nonnegotiable value. From this follows that the only morally justifiable reason for withholding or withdrawing life-prolonging medical treatment would be the conviction that such treatment cannot be useful or effective.

Voluntary euthanasia: See **euthanasia**

$\backsim\mathbf{W}\backsim$

Washington v. Glucksberg: 1997 U.S. Supreme Court (521 U.S. 702 [1997]) case regarding the question of a constitutional right to assistance in **suicide.** The laws of the State of Washington prohibited assisted suicide but specified that withholding or withdrawing life-prolonging treatment was not suicide but rather a matter of respecting individual rights to refuse unwanted treatment. Petitioners claimed that Washington's legal restrictions upon one's freedom to seek assistance in committing suicide violate "liberty interests" protected by the due process clause of the Fourteenth Amendment of the U.S. Constitution. The Supreme Court majority held, however, that "the 'right' to assistance in committing suicide is not a fundamental liberty interest protected by the Due Process Clause." Furthermore, the Court held that the Washington law was "rationally related" to legitimate state interests, including the preservation of human life, the public health concern for preventing suicide, protection of the "integrity and ethics of the medical profession," protecting vulnerable groups from abuse or coercion, and preventing a **slippery slope** toward voluntary or involuntary **euthanasia.** (See also *Vacco v. Quill,* another case regarding the right to assisted suicide decided by the Supreme Court on the same day.)

Wedge argument: See **slippery slope argument**.

Withholding and withdrawing (life-prolonging treatment): An often-discussed differentiation based in a sense of moral difference between not instituting a form of treatment that

185

will prolong life on the one hand and removing or withdrawing a treatment that is currently prolonging life on the other. Certainly, health care providers often experience a psychological difference between the two: When life-prolonging treatment is withheld, the "natural" trajectory of the patient's anticipated death from underlying disease or injury is simply not interrupted; but when treatment that is currently sustaining life is withdrawn, then that removal itself is perceived to be the "cause" of subsequent decline and death of the patient (often in a short period of time). However, many philosophers, theologians, judicial courts, health care organizations, and provider associations agree that there is little, if any, moral or legal distinction to be drawn between decisions to withhold or to withdraw life-prolonging treatment per se. In either case a pathology (disease or injury) will, without treatment intervention, clearly cause the patient's death. The only human choice to be made is whether medical or surgical interventions will be used to compensate for the effects of that pathology and thus forestall death at least temporarily. If, then, good moral reasons exist for choosing not to forestall death by initiating life-sustaining treatments (see **"extraordinary" and "ordinary" means of treatment),** the same reasons would justify a decision to cease forestalling death via life-sustaining treatments. (See, e.g., American Medical Association Council on Ethical and Judicial Affairs, "Decisions near the End of Life," *JAMA* 267 no. 16 [April 22/29, 1992]: 2229–33.)

Wrongful birth: In tort law, a form of medical malpractice claim in which the parents of a child born with birth defects allege that misdiagnosis or negligent treatment or advice from a physician deprived them of the opportunity to avoid that child's birth by terminating the pregnancy (or in some cases preventing conception). In most wrongful birth cases, the parents of the child born with defects seek damages based on the costs (to them) of having to raise a child with unexpected disabilities. Only a minority of U.S. state courts explicitly recognize the validity of wrongful birth actions.

Wrongful life: In tort law, a form of medical malpractice claim brought on behalf of a child born with birth defects that alleges, essentially, the child would be better off not having been born in her condition and was born only due to misdiagnosis of that condition or negligent advice or treatment of the parent(s). In most instances, a wrongful life claim seeks damages from a physician or hospital based (in theory) upon the burdens the child must bear living with her disabilities. Only a small number of states permit wrongful life actions, in large part because a finding of wrongful life requires acceptance of the premise that being born with a disability is indeed worse than not being born at all, and that such a comparison could actually be made. In its most extreme form, a few wrongful life claims have been pressed on behalf of a child against her parents (alleging that the parents were accurately informed of the diagnosed defects or disabilities and chose to continue with the pregnancy, thus allowing a worse-than-death outcome for their child). None of these latter cases has ever been successful to date.

✄ X ✄

Xenograft: Organ or tissue transplanted from one individual to another individual of another species. (See **transplantation, organ and tissue**)

Xenotransplantation: Removal of organ or tissue from an individual of one species and implantation of that tissue into an individual of another species. (See **transplantation, organ and tissue**)

X-linked recessive disorders: Genetic disorders or diseases caused by a **mutation** on the X chromosome. (Males have inherited an X and a Y chromosome while females have inherited two X chromosomes, one from each parent.) X-linked recessive disorders are manifest in the male if he carries the mutated form of the X chromosome in his cells but are manifest in the female only if she inherited the mutated form of the X chromosome from both parents. (See **disorder, genetic**)

~Z~

ZIFT: See **zygote intrafallopian transfer**

Zona pellucida: The membrane that forms around an **ovum** as it develops in the female ovary. At fertilization, the sperm must penetrate the zona pellucida to combine the chromosomal contents of egg and sperm. After fertilization, the zona pellucida gradually disappears to facilitate implantation of the fertilized ovum into the lining of the uterus.

Zygote: The cell resulting from the fertilization of an ovum by a sperm cell. (See **embryonic development**)

Zygote intrafallopian transfer (ZIFT): An assisted reproductive technology in which fertilization of ova by sperm is allowed to happen in a laboratory dish, after which the resulting zygotes (pre embryos) are transferred to the woman's fallopian tube (through which they will travel to the uterus for implantation). (See **assisted reproductive technology**)